• LIVING WELL WITH ORTHOSTATIC INTOLERANCE •

LIVING WELL WITH

ORTHO STATIC INTOLERANCE

A Guide to Diagnosis and Treatment

PETER C. ROWE, MD

JOHNS HOPKINS UNIVERSITY PRESS | *Baltimore*

Johns Hopkins University Press
2715 North Charles Street
Baltimore, Maryland 21218
www.press.jhu.edu

Library of Congress Cataloging-in-Publication Data is available.

A catalog record for this book is available from the British Library.

ISBN 978-1-4214-4942-5 (hardcover)
ISBN 978-1-4214-5025-4 (paperback)
ISBN 978-1-4214-5026-1 (ebook)

A catalog record for this book is available from the British Library.

Special discounts are available for bulk purchases of this book. For more information, please contact Special Sales at specialsales@jh.edu.

CONTENTS

ABBREVIATIONS

ADH	antidiuretic hormone
ANS	autonomic nervous system
BMI	body mass index
BP	blood pressure
bpm	beats per minute
CBC	complete blood count
CMP	comprehensive metabolic panel
CMV	cytomegalovirus
cOH	classical orthostatic hypotension
dOH	delayed orthostatic hypotension
ECG	electrocardiogram
EDS	Ehlers–Danlos syndrome
ESR	erythrocyte sedimentation rate
HCN	hyperpolarization-activated cyclic nucleotide
HR	heart rate
iOH	initial orthostatic hypotension
IST	inappropriate sinus tachycardia
IV	intravenous
MALS	median arcuate ligament syndrome

MCAS	mast cell activation syndrome
MCV	mean corpuscular volume
ME/CFS	myalgic encephalomyelitis/chronic fatigue syndrome
mg	milligram
mL	milliliter
mm Hg	millimeters of mercury
MRI	magnetic resonance imaging
NMH	neurally mediated hypotension
NSAID	nonsteroidal anti-inflammatory drug
nTOS	neurogenic thoracic outlet syndrome
OH	orthostatic hypotension
POTS	postural tachycardia syndrome
RDW	red cell distribution width
SNRI	serotonin–norepinephrine reuptake inhibitor
SSRI	selective serotonin reuptake inhibitor

PREFACE

Orthostatic: relating to or caused by an upright posture.
—Oxford English Dictionary

Orthostatic intolerance describes a group of circulatory disorders in which symptoms are brought on by quiet upright posture and are largely alleviated by lying down. In the early 1990s, intrigued by how commonly orthostatic intolerance affected our patients with chronic fatigue, I began putting together a practical guide on how to manage orthostatic intolerance syndromes. Over the past three decades, this guide has been improved upon by input from our patients and their families as well as my health care colleagues.

The principles of managing orthostatic intolerance described in this book emerge from those efforts and apply to a wide group of circulatory conditions, including neurally mediated hypotension, recurrent syncope, orthostatic hypotension, and postural tachycardia syndrome. They also apply to individuals with symptoms of orthostatic intolerance but no clear heart rate or blood pressure abnormalities. The book should also be helpful to those with disorders in which these circulatory problems are prominent, including myalgic encephalomyelitis/chronic fatigue syndrome (ME/CFS), fibromyalgia, Ehlers–Danlos syndrome, other conditions characterized by joint hypermobility, postinfectious fatigue (including Lyme disease and post-COVID-19 conditions/long COVID), postcancer fatigue, and even some forms of fatigue that affect athletes with inconsistent training and performance.

While primarily written to help patients and families, the book includes details on medication dosing and a reference list, so physicians, nurses, physical therapists, and other health care team members should also find it helpful. Because the majority of our clinic patients have ME/CFS, and the vast majority of ME/CFS patients have orthostatic intolerance, many of our examples mention this disorder but also apply to other conditions. While orthostatic intolerance is not universal in ME/CFS, it is found in over 95% of pediatric ME/CFS patients, and recent work shows that it also affects 90% of adults with the disorder.

Because some of the words we use may be unfamiliar to nonmedical readers, we use bold font to identify terms defined in the glossary at the end of the book.

I would especially like to thank Katherine Lucas and Elly Brosius for sharing their insights on ME/CFS as we began working on this condition in the early 1990s. I also want to thank all those whose work is reflected in these pages, including Dr. Kevin Kelly in pediatric gastroenterology, Rick Violand and Scott Heinlein in physical therapy, my cardiology collaborators including Dr. Hugh Calkins and Dr. Issam Bou-Holaigah at Johns Hopkins, and Dr. Linda Van Campen and Dr. Frans Visser in the Netherlands. We have benefited from the expertise of my geneticist colleagues, including Dr. Michael Geraghty and Dr. Clair Francomano, and from our surgical colleagues, Dr. Daniel Heffez, Dr. Charles Edwards II, and Dr. Fraser Henderson. My research coordinator Colleen Marden and occupational therapist

Samantha Jasion helped with the first draft of turning the earlier brochure into a more detailed version. Lindsay Petracek, BSc, was the driving force who worked diligently with me in the last year to revise and format the current book. We thank Colleen Marden; Renee Swope, RN; Carla Rowe; Dr. Camille Broussard; and Meghan Swope for their comments and suggestions on the manuscript.

Our Chronic Fatigue Clinic at the Johns Hopkins Children's Center would not have been possible without the incredible philanthropic support we have received over the past 30 years. I want to single out for special recognition The Sunshine Natural Wellbeing Foundation, which provided the funds for an endowed professorship that has allowed me to continue working on research and education activities. Bill and Vicki Boies have been generous and consistent supporters over the past 25 years, as have Jean and Steve Caldwell. They and the other donors to the CFS program have provided me the freedom to continue seeing complex patients without the time constraints we often face in modern medicine. We are fortunate to have been supported by other families too numerous to mention here but whose contributions have been vital. They all deserve a share in whatever credit the program has achieved.

Peter C. Rowe, MD
Professor of Pediatrics
Sunshine Natural Wellbeing Foundation Professor of Chronic Fatigue and Related Disorders
Division of Adolescent and Young Adult Medicine
The Johns Hopkins University School of Medicine
Baltimore 2023

Introduction

My fatigue is constant, worse with even modest exertion, such as carrying the grocery bags or walking around the block. On a good day, if I tend to do more, I get worse symptoms for the next two to three days. After watching my son's baseball game, I had to recline for much of the next two days. I have to limit the number of errands I perform each day, often to just one trip out of the house, and I can't do the same activity two days in a row without getting worse fatigue and much more difficulty concentrating. I am more exhausted, lightheaded, and mentally foggy when standing in line or sitting for long periods. I get really lightheaded in the shower and have to lie down for 20 minutes afterwards to recover.
—Elizabeth Kastor, patient

Orthostatic intolerance refers to a group of circulatory disorders in which symptoms are brought on by quiet upright posture and are largely alleviated by lying down. A common problem in the field of medicine, it can contribute to impaired quality of life and reduced activity. Symptoms include chronic lightheadedness, fatigue, and difficulty thinking and concentrating. Despite its prevalence, it was a relatively neglected area of medicine in the last century. In the days before the development of effective therapies for **hypertension** (high blood pressure), the *New England Journal of Medicine* published a paper titled "Hypotension: the ideal normal blood pressure."[1] To propose that **hypotension** (low blood pressure) is optimal might have been a reasonable claim in the 1940s before the advent of effective treatment, especially given the high levels of morbidity and mortality (including heart attacks and strokes) caused by untreated, chronically elevated blood pressure. Now that we have better treatments, it is no longer reasonable to make this assertion. In fact, doing so involves ignoring the sometimes disabling symptoms that can accompany low blood pressure and other forms of orthostatic intolerance.

Medical attention to disorders associated with chronic fatigue began to emerge after the US Civil War and after World War I, as a number of soldiers developed incapacitating illnesses characterized by exhaustion. By the 1940s, several groups drew attention to the possibility that these fatiguing disorders were associated with abnormal control of blood circulation.[2] Two military physicians, Alexander MacLean and Edgar Allen, described several patients who experienced orthostatic **tachycardia** (an excessive heart rate [HR] acceleration) and a drop in blood pressure after moving from the recumbent to the upright posture. This was usually associated with symptoms of orthostatic exhaustion, weakness during exercise, blurred vision, and **syncope** (fainting). MacLean and Allen held that the increased heart rate was a response to a reduced return of venous blood to the heart from the lower half of the body. Using the synonyms of the day, they concluded that this orthostatic tachycardia and hypotension syndrome seemed identical with what we now call *myalgic encephalomyelitis/chronic fatigue syndrome* (ME/CFS). In their early reports, MacLean and Allen described improvement in patients after increased fluid and salt intake. Despite these pioneering observations, their work was largely ignored for several decades.

By the 1980s, more attention was directed to these circulatory problems. In the 1990s, it began to emerge that orthostatic intolerance could accompany a variety of chronic conditions, including ME/CFS, fibromyalgia, Ehlers–Danlos syndrome, and other disorders in which fatigue was a prominent symptom. Research has described different types of heart rate and blood pressure responses to upright posture, including postural tachycardia syndrome (POTS), neurally mediated hypotension (NMH), and others. This field is still relatively young, and a complete consensus about the optimal approach to and treatment for orthostatic intolerance eludes us. This book, based on our experience at the Johns Hopkins Hospital, provides guidance on living with and managing these disorders, drawing on the scientific evidence where it is available and on our clinical understandings when it is not. Although older individuals with orthostatic disorders like those that accompany Parkinson's disease and other degenerative neurological conditions might find this book's suggestions helpful, we focus on the forms of orthostatic intolerance that affect individuals from adolescence to middle age.

Chapter 1 describes in greater detail how the autonomic nervous system orchestrates the normal and abnormal circulatory responses to upright posture. The symptoms associated with the abnormal responses—as observed by MacLean and Allen—are discussed in chapter 2. The autonomic nervous system is responsible for multiple changes in bodily function beyond the control of circulation, including pupillary size, sweating, digestion and movement of food through the intestinal tract, bladder emptying, and temperature regulation. When the autonomic control of circulation is impaired, it is not surprising that individuals can experience a myriad of symptoms throughout the body. These other forms of dysautonomia (dysfunction of the autonomic nervous system) will not be the primary focus of this book, but it is important to acknowledge that orthostatic intolerance can occur in conjunction with widespread symptoms.

In chapter 3, we discuss how the diagnosis of orthostatic intolerance is typically made with an in-office passive standing test or a more formal head-up tilt table test. Orthostatic intolerance can be triggered by infectious illnesses or by surgery and trauma. We assume, throughout the book, that patients reporting fatigue and other orthostatic symptoms will have been evaluated by their physicians to ensure that other medical causes, from the mundane (e.g., sleep deprivation) to the critical (e.g., leukemia), will have been identified by standard clinical care. Because other disorders may not be recognizable at an early point, it is imperative to remain observant for other causes of symptoms while initiating treatment of the orthostatic disorder. Orthostatic intolerance can accompany nearly any other chronic medical illness and can occasionally be prominent in those with primarily psychiatric disorders, such as anorexia nervosa or bulimia. Focusing on the orthostatic intolerance and failing to recognize the eating disorder could have fatal consequences. Conversely, in the past, individuals with orthostatic intolerance and chronic fatigue had been viewed as having primarily **psychosomatic** conditions based on an erroneous judgment that the physical examination and laboratory values were normal. One medical historian claimed that our culture was witnessing a "kind of collective hypervigilance about the body" and a "readiness of a large number of people to cling tenaciously to a given diagnosis [ME/CFS], refusing to abandon their belief despite medical reassurance to the contrary."[3] The medical reassurance at the time, namely that there was nothing physically wrong with people who had ME/CFS, proved to be incorrect, largely because no one was testing for orthostatic intolerance. Patients who correctly felt that there was something wrong were caught in a Catch-22: the more they expressed this belief, the more it was seen as "protesting too much" and misinterpreted as further evidence of a psychosomatic condition. Our research and clinical work since 1995 draws a different conclusion, as does much of the subsequent research by others, moving us to a different vantage point in considering these chronic disorders. Old ideas linger, however, and our approach is not shared by all.

After diagnosis, the treatment of orthostatic intolerance requires a mix of dietary and lifestyle changes, along with judicious use of medications. Chapters 4–6 review the common nonpharmacologic therapies that can improve function, including a higher sodium intake, compression garments, physical countermaneuvers that use the leg muscles to pump the blood back up to the heart and brain, and manual physical therapy techniques. We also describe the importance of treating comorbid (coexisting) medical conditions that can influence tolerance of upright posture. Chapter 6 provides detailed guidance about the commonly used medications that treat orthostatic intolerance for those whose symptoms persist despite conservative management.

In chapter 7, we bring the overall approach into greater focus by describing the course of several patients from the clinic. This illustrates some of the differences between patients regarding symptoms and outcomes. For instructional purposes, we have selected stories of patients who improved, but this does not suggest that the course is always as straightforward or successful. The management of orthostatic intolerance requires patience and perseverance on the parts of affected individuals, their families, and their healthcare teams. We anticipate further advances to emerge from the continued scientific study of this group of problems, but as we await those insights, affected patients need assistance now, and it would be grossly unfair to ask them to wait years for the results from randomized clinical trials.

CHAPTER 1

Basics of Orthostatic Intolerance

The first example of orthostatic intolerance that I can remember was in kindergarten, standing on the back row of bleachers during a concert. I was terrified that I would fall off the back of the bleachers. I couldn't understand why nobody else had the same fear. Thirteen years later, when I got diagnosed with POTS and NMH, I finally realized that fear had been because I got dizzy and lightheaded and was having signs of orthostatic intolerance. Of course, five-year-old me didn't know what dizziness and lightheadedness were, so how was I supposed to let my parents and teachers know that? Years later, I'm still discovering symptoms that I thought were normal that actually aren't.

—Lindsay Petracek, patient

The medical term *orthostatic* is defined as relating to or being caused by an upright posture. *Orthostatic intolerance*, then, is an umbrella term for several conditions in which symptoms are worsened by assuming and maintaining an upright posture. This most commonly refers to standing, but prolonged sitting can also provoke symptoms. Many of these orthostatic symptoms improve with lying down, but once provoked, some symptoms—such as fatigue and brain fog—can persist for hours. Lightheadedness, in contrast, usually improves promptly upon assuming a recumbent position.

Circulation depends on the heart to pump blood through the arteries and into smaller arterioles and capillaries. On the arterial side of the circulation, oxygen, carried by hemoglobin in the red blood cells, passes into progressively smaller vessels in all body tissues. Oxygen and nutrients diffuse into cells, enabling optimal cellular function. The venous side of the circulation is a lower-pressure circuit that removes waste products from cells and returns blood to the right side of the heart. From there, blood is pumped into the lungs to pick up oxygen and return to the left side of the heart.[1] The entire process is regulated by the autonomic nervous system (ANS), which controls the involuntary, or automatic, components of the nervous system, such as blood pressure and breathing.

The ANS is comprised of the parasympathetic division (which originates from the brainstem and the lower spinal cord) and the sympathetic division (which originates from the mid-spinal cord), which work together to help the body maintain homeostasis (a stable internal environment). When external conditions change, the body must adjust its internal environment. For example, when we are cold (external environment), the ANS constricts blood vessels in our extremities to keep our organs warm (internal environment). Without this ANS response, our vital organs would get cold too, and they would not function properly. When we stand up too quickly (external environment), the ANS increases our blood pressure (internal environment) to keep us from fainting. In order to adjust our body's internal environment, the parasympathetic and sympathetic divisions have opposing functions. For example, the parasympathetic division slows the heart rate, and the sympathetic division accelerates it.[2]

These examples are oversimplifications. The responses involve a chain reaction of multiple events across many parts of the body. External changes can cause internal changes, which activate the ANS. The nerves can sense environmental changes and send messages to other nerves via pathways (neural circuits), telling the body how to respond. If part of a neural circuit does not receive or send a message correctly, it can cause the parasympathetic and sympathetic divisions to over- or underreact. This does not always mean that there is a problem with the ANS. For example, upon standing with low blood volume, receptors tell the ANS that there is not enough blood going to vital organs and it needs to increase sympathetic activity, which causes an increase in the heart rate and blood pressure. In this case, the change is not due to a problem with the ANS but to the low blood volume.

Orthostatic intolerance is sometimes referred to as *dysautonomia*—a dysfunction of the autonomic nervous system. While orthostatic intolerance can be a symptom of dysautonomia, not all forms of dysautonomia involve orthostatic intolerance. For example, excessive sweating is governed by the ANS, and while it is often associated with orthostatic intolerance, it can occur independently of circulatory dysregulation. Similarly, problems with slow intestinal transit can be caused by dysautonomia but are not necessarily associated with orthostatic intolerance.

Normal and Abnormal Responses to Upright Posture

When a healthy individual stands up, gravity causes 10–15% of blood to settle in the abdomen, arms, and legs.[3] This pooling of blood means that less blood returns to the heart and less reaches the brain. To compensate, the body turns on a series of rapid reflex responses that increase the release of **norepinephrine** and **epinephrine** (also known as noradrenaline and adrenaline, respectively). Both substances typically cause the heart to beat a little faster and with more force (a familiar feeling after we exercise or are frightened). In addition, norepinephrine constricts the blood vessels. The result is more blood returning to the heart and brain. Most of the time, we are unaware of these reflex changes in blood flow when we stand up.

When people with orthostatic intolerance are upright, they appear to pool a larger amount of blood in vessels below heart level than healthy individuals. The longer they remain upright, the greater the proportion of blood that settles in their abdomen and limbs. Along with increased blood pooling, many individuals with orthostatic intolerance syndromes have a lower-than-normal amount of blood in the circulation. The lower blood volume becomes more important if the individual is not drinking adequate amounts of fluid or is losing body fluids due to vomiting, diarrhea, excessive sweating, or increased urination. In response to increased pooling, lower blood volume, or both, the body releases more norepinephrine or epinephrine when the person with orthostatic intolerance is upright. For a variety of reasons, not all of which are well understood, the vessels do not seem to respond normally to these substances, and they either do not constrict efficiently or they dilate. Because the heart remains able to respond to the norepinephrine and epinephrine, the heart rate often increases.

Figure 1-1 shows the main influences on the ability to remain free of symptoms (asymptomatic) when upright in those with orthostatic intolerance. In those with postural tachycardia syndrome (POTS), the main result of excessive blood pooling during upright posture is an exaggerated rise in heart rate.[4] In those with neurally mediated hypotension (NMH), the main result is a reflex lowering of blood pressure

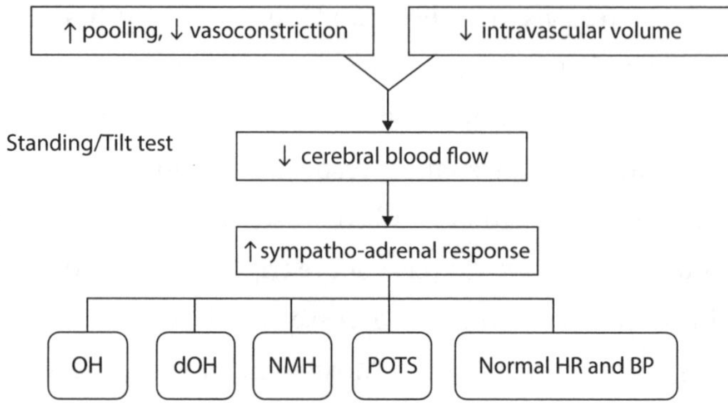

Figure 1-1. The main pathophysiological influences on orthostatic intolerance. Abbreviations: OH (orthostatic hypotension); dOH (delayed OH); NMH (neurally mediated hypotension); POTS (postural tachycardia syndrome); HR (heart rate); and BP (blood pressure).

(BP).[5] Some of this is caused by a "miscommunication" between the heart and brain, both of which are usually structurally normal. Just when the heart needs to beat faster to pump blood to the brain and prevent fainting, the brain tells it to beat slower and the blood vessels to dilate further. These actions take even more blood away from where it is needed in the central part of the circulation. At this time, it is not entirely clear why people develop different forms of orthostatic intolerance, although some researchers believe it may relate, in part, to the balance of epinephrine and norepinephrine release.[6]

One of the physical signs often present in those with orthostatic intolerance syndromes is a reddish-purple discoloration most evident in the hands and feet when upright. The medical term for this is **acrocyanosis** (*acro* means extremity; *cyanosis* refers to skin discoloration usually seen when there is a higher concentration of hemoglobin that no longer carries as much oxygen).[7] Figure 1-2 shows an example of acrocyanosis in a 19-year-old college student who described lightheadedness and fatigue. Her symptoms were worse with exposure to hot baths, hot weather, increased physical exertion, shopping, and menstrual periods. We evaluated her with a 10-minute standing test. The left side of Figure 1-2 shows the degree of acrocyanosis in her hand after five minutes of the test, with a healthy individual's hand behind hers for contrast. The right side of the figure shows where the examiner had compressed the skin of her lower leg. Over the next six to eight seconds, after picking up a camera, focusing it, and taking the picture, she still had a lack of blood return to the compressed areas, a phenomenon known as *delayed capillary refill*. We interpret the acrocyanosis, in part, as a reflection of the increased blood pooling in the dependent limbs and, in general, as a sign of the abnormal blood circulation in these conditions. Acrocyanosis is not always present in those with orthostatic intolerance, but in some individuals, it can be quite dramatic, extending above the knee.

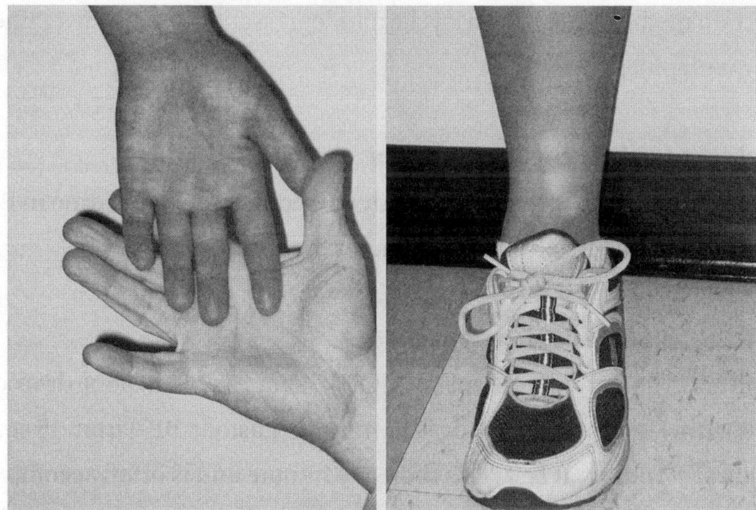

Figure 1-2. Acrocyanosis. Both panels show the discoloration of the skin in the dependent limbs. On the right, the examiner has compressed the skin, and there has been almost no capillary refill (blood return) to the compressed areas after more than five seconds (normal capillary refill occurs within three seconds).

Definitions of Different Forms of Orthostatic Intolerance

As illustrated in Figure 1-1, there are multiple categories of orthostatic intolerance, often defined by the heart rate and blood pressure responses. **Systolic blood pressure** refers to the pressure in the arteries when the heart's ventricles contract, and **diastolic blood pressure** refers to the pressure when the ventricles relax and refill. Blood pressure is usually measured in millimeters of mercury (mm Hg).

Classical Orthostatic Hypotension

Classical orthostatic hypotension (cOH) requires a sustained drop of 20 mm Hg in systolic BP or a drop of 10 mm Hg in diastolic BP within the first three minutes of standing or head-up tilt.[8] This condition is more common in older adults but can be seen in younger individuals experiencing acute dehydration, anorexia nervosa, or a response to certain medications (e.g., tricyclic antidepressants, prochlorperazine, or quetiapine).

Delayed Orthostatic Hypotension

Delayed orthostatic hypotension (dOH) requires the same drop in BP as cOH but occurs after three minutes upright.

Initial Orthostatic Hypotension

Initial orthostatic hypotension (iOH) requires a transient drop of > 40 mm Hg in systolic BP or > 20 mm Hg diastolic BP within 15 seconds of standing. It lasts less than one minute and is often accompanied by lightheadedness and reflex tachycardia.[9] iOH is common in adolescents. It does not require treatment if there are no chronic daily symptoms that interfere with normal function. Syncope is uncommon. iOH can be associated with postural tachycardia syndrome.[10]

Neurally Mediated Hypotension

Neurally mediated hypotension (NMH) requires a reflex drop in BP after being upright. It is sometimes known as *reflex syncope, neurocardiogenic syncope*, or *vasovagal syncope*.[11] We prefer the term *neurally mediated hypotension* because many people with this response during tilt table testing do not have recurrent syncope in day-to-day life. We define NMH as a drop in systolic BP of 25 mm Hg during standing or upright tilt table testing compared to the BP when the person is lying flat.[12] It is often accompanied by slowing of the heart rate (**bradycardia**) at the time of hypotension. NMH is the most common cause of syncope at all ages, more commonly in women and adolescents. Although it may be slightly more common in people with a low resting BP, most people who develop NMH during standing have a normal resting BP. NMH is an abnormality in BP regulation with upright posture when too little blood circulates back to the heart, a situation that can trigger an abnormal reflex interaction between the heart and the brain that results in a BP drop. Although some physicians write that patients with NMH identified during tilt table testing only have syncope and are fine between fainting episodes, our experience is that this physiology can cause chronic daily symptoms.

Figure 1-3 shows the patterns of BP and heart rate response during orthostatic testing in two individuals with NMH. The upper panel shows the response of a young medical student who reported recurrent daily lightheadedness, daily fatigue, and difficulty thinking and concentrating, made worse by sitting in class for most of the day. She had a nine beat-per-minute (bpm) increase in her heart rate immediately after being raised to a 70° head-up angle on the tilt table test, associated with reproduction of her lightheadedness and pallor. At the six-minute point, she suddenly developed a sharp drop in heart rate and BP, with her BP falling to 50 mm Hg—a pressure inconsistent with remaining conscious. She developed some brief seizure activity, which

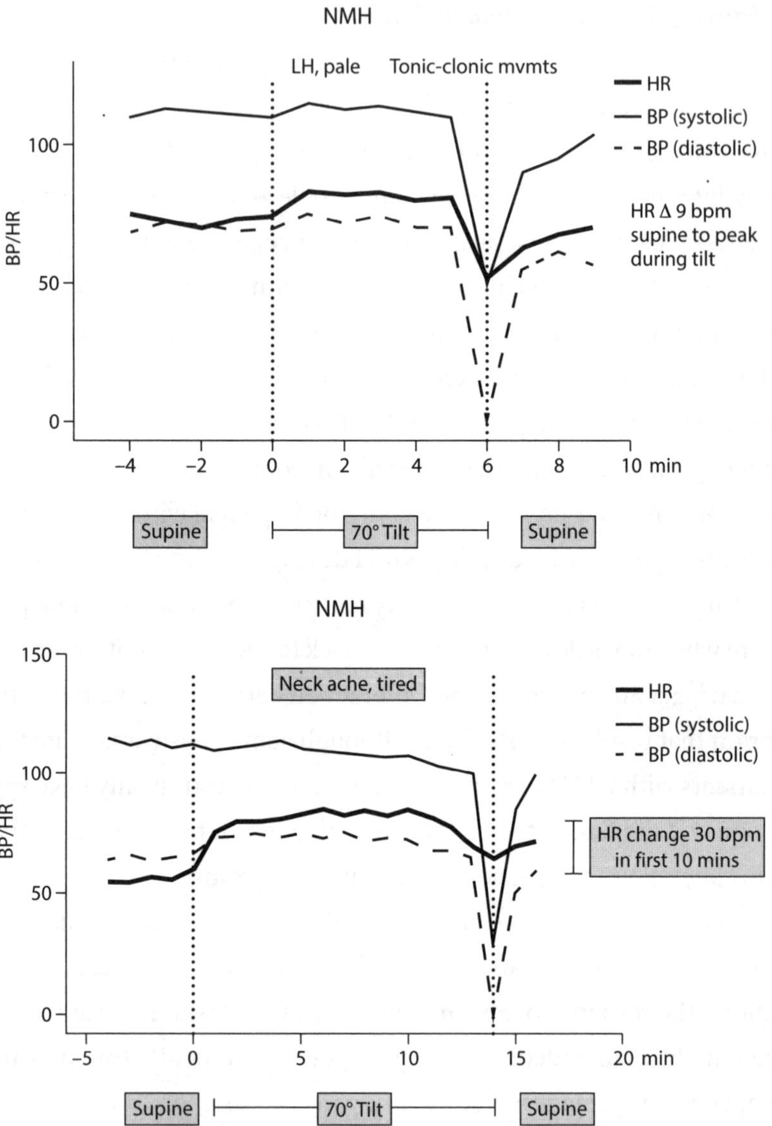

Figure 1-3. Standing and tilt table test results in individuals with neurally mediated hypotension. Abbreviations: LH (lightheaded) and mvmts (movements).

sometimes accompanies the abrupt reduction in brain blood flow when this reflex pattern occurs. The onset of the BP reduction in those with NMH is often closer to 30 minutes into the tilt test, but as demonstrated in this young medical student, it can occur at an early point.

On the lower panel of Figure 1-3 is the tilt table response of a 16-year-old adolescent with chronic fatigue, lightheadedness, neck pain, upper back pain, and difficulty concentrating. She had a modest 30-bpm increase in heart rate in the first 10 minutes of upright tilt, associated with reproduction of her typical symptoms. This was followed by the same abrupt drop in BP and an associated reduction in heart rate at the 14-minute point.

Postural Tachycardia Syndrome (POTS)

POTS is characterized by an exaggerated increase in heart rate with standing along with chronic orthostatic symptoms.[13] A healthy individual usually has a slight increase in heart rate—10–20 bpm—within the first 10 minutes of standing. POTS occurs when the heart rate increases by ≥ 30 bpm for adults (ages ≥ 20) or ≥ 40 bpm for adolescents (ages 12–19). There are no set criteria for children under the age of 12, although some committees apply the 40-bpm criteria to children as young as 6 years old. Single elevations of heart rate—especially in the first minute—that are not followed by substantial heart rate increases should not be classified as POTS. In general, the heart rate elevation should be sustained during the orthostatic stress, although definitions of POTS lack specific guidance regarding the duration. One example where experts might disagree is a case in which a 19-year-old develops a 30-bpm rise initially on standing, then has a further gradual increase to a peak heart rate increment of 40 bpm at the 10-minute point. This individual meets the heart rate increment criteria for POTS, but does this qualify as sustained? Subsequent refinement of the POTS criteria may clarify how patients should be classified under this rubric.

POTS must be accompanied by chronic orthostatic symptoms. Symptoms of POTS and other forms of orthostatic intolerance can be provoked by prolonged quiet sitting, although the usual emphasis is on the more rapid onset of symptoms with standing. POTS is an abnormality in the regulation of heart rate; most commonly, the heart itself is structurally normal. Some patients with POTS, in the first 10 minutes of upright standing or tilt testing, will go on to develop NMH if the test is continued; the two conditions can be found together and are not mutually exclusive.

The upper panel of Figure 1-4 shows an adolescent female whose resting heart rate was normal but increased rapidly as soon as she stood up. As she remained in a quiet standing position, without shifting her weight or fidgeting, her heart rate increased from 62 bpm to 113 bpm—a remarkable 51-bpm change—associated with increased lightheadedness, fatigue, and nausea. This is a classic example of POTS in adolescence. The lower panel in Figure 1-4 illustrates an early 44-bpm increase in heart rate in the first 10 minutes of tilt table testing, followed by the development of an NMH response abruptly at the 20-minute point. Stopping the test after just 10 minutes would have missed the drop in BP.

Some experts prefer to distinguish between subtypes of POTS, including neuropathic, hypovolemic, and hyperadrenergic forms. These categories are based on the pathophysiologic mechanisms described earlier in the chapter. We would emphasize that the subtypes overlap, and most patients have some degree of reduced blood volume. All forms involve some degree of hyperadrenergic response to the reduction in brain blood flow when individuals are upright.

The neuropathic subtype is characterized by partial autonomic neuropathy (some of the nerves that control autonomic functions do

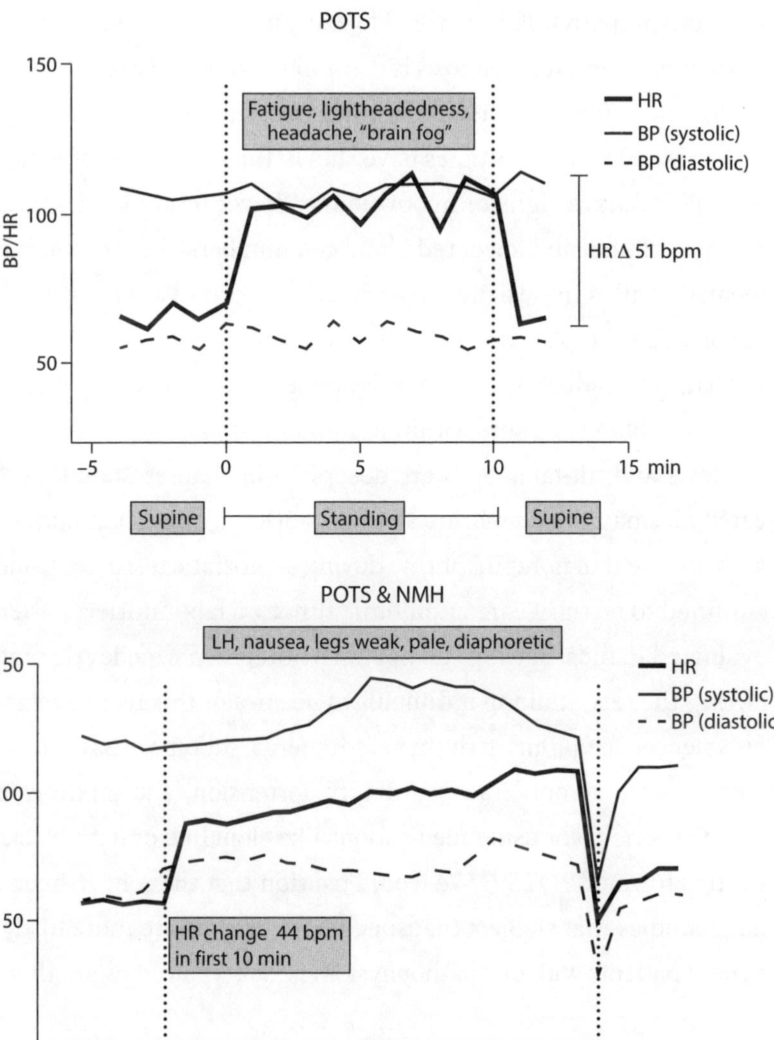

Figure 1-4. Standing and tilt test results in individuals with postural tachycardia syndrome (POTS), one of whom developed neurally mediated hypotension (NMH) beyond the first 10 minutes upright.

not work properly). This can lead to excessive venous pooling during upright posture. Acrocyanosis is common in this subtype.

As the name suggests, the hypovolemic subtype is characterized by low blood volume. Studies have shown that up to 70% of patients with POTS have signs of hypovolemia (lower total blood volume, plasma volume, and lower red blood cell numbers), but this does not mean that all of these patients would be categorized as having the hypovolemic subtype.

The hyperadrenergic subtype is defined by a $\geq$ 20 mm Hg increase in systolic blood pressure within 10 minutes of standing or tilt (standing tests and tilt-table tests are described in chapter 3) and an elevated plasma norepinephrine level of $\geq$ 600 pg/mL when upright.[14] Measurement of norepinephrine during orthostatic testing is usually confined to tertiary care autonomic function laboratories. Patients evaluated in most settings do not have norepinephrine levels drawn during the test, making it difficult to be sure of this form's relative prevalence. Symptoms in the hyperadrenergic subtype usually include palpitations, tremors, tachycardia, hypertension, and anxiety, and some experts favor using medications like clonidine or beta-blockers for this form of POTS.[15] We would caution that there have been no large studies that suggest that specific treatments are more likely to benefit patients with one pathophysiologic subtype versus another.

Inappropriate Sinus Tachycardia

Inappropriate sinus tachycardia (IST) requires a resting heart rate greater than 100 bpm. The symptoms are similar to those of POTS.[16]

Low Orthostatic Tolerance

Low orthostatic tolerance is the presence of orthostatic symptoms without meeting criteria for cOH, dOH, NMH, IST, or POTS. For many with low orthostatic tolerance, the symptoms are due to a reduction in **cerebral blood flow**. As an example, approximately 60% of adults with ME/CFS have a normal BP and heart rate response to 30 minutes of head-up tilt testing. When upright for the same period of time, healthy individuals have an approximately 7% reduction in cerebral blood flow compared to their supine values. ME/CFS patients who have no evidence of POTS or hypotension have, on average, a 24% reduction in cerebral blood flow when upright, even though values are equal to those of healthy individuals when supine.[17] People with low orthostatic tolerance can have just as many symptoms, often with similar severity, as those with POTS and NMH. The cerebral blood flow reductions can occur with lesser degrees of orthostatic stress than a full 30-minute 70° upright tilt table test. In more severely affected patients, a 20° upright angle of the tilt-test or just sitting in a chair can provoke similar > 20% reductions in brain blood flow.[18]

CHAPTER 2

Symptoms

I used to empty and fill the dishwasher, change the sheets on my bed, put away my clothes, as some of my responsibilities. Now, each of these activities triggers tachycardia (POTS episodes).

For a long time, I thought it was normal to have to crouch down in the shower, and then lay on the floor after a shower, because of a pounding, rapid heartbeat that exhausts me and leaves my brain even more fogged. I used to attend school full-time, participate in theater and swim competitively. Now, I am housebound. I can leave the house no more than twice a week for physical therapy without overwhelming payback afterwards.

I **want** to be more active.

I **want** to be able to hang out with people.

I **want** to be able to go to school.

I want to be **MYSELF** again.

—testimony from Alexander Lopez-Majano at the US Health and Human Services Chronic Fatigue Syndrome Advisory Committee meeting, Fall 2010

When the brain receives too little blood flow, the usual result is a light-headed or spacey feeling. Some people describe this as a "head rush." Others notice that they feel generally unwell or tired when standing still, without specifically endorsing lightheadedness. Recurrent lightheadedness is a common symptom of orthostatic intolerance. If lightheadedness is severe, individuals can develop dimmed vision, distorted hearing, nausea, or vomiting. They might faint because not enough blood is getting to the brain. Fainting is helpful in that it restores a person to a horizontal position, removing the effect of gravity on blood pooling in the limbs and allowing more blood to return to the heart. Following the episodes of lightheadedness or fainting, most people feel tired for several hours (sometimes more than a day), an observation that dates back to the early part of the 20th century.[1] Their thinking can be somewhat foggy. Some patients experience prolonged fatigue and other symptoms (termed **postexertional malaise**) after a modest amount of physical activity, after sustained quiet activity like sitting at a desk, or after prolonged standing. This post-exertional malaise can last beyond 24–72 hours and can interfere with daily activities.

It is worth emphasizing that while fainting has been considered a classic symptom of NMH, we have found that many people who develop NMH during tilt table testing do not faint in day-to-day life.[2] Chronic fatigue, muscle aches (also termed **myalgias**), headaches, nausea, and problems with thinking can be prominent symptoms of NMH in these individuals. The cognitive symptoms can take the form of difficulty concentrating, staying on task, paying attention, processing what is going on, remembering, or finding the right words. Some describe a sense of "brain fog."[3] Some develop worse fatigue after mentally demanding activities, such as reading and concentrating. This might occur because the blood vessels of the limbs dilate rather than constrict in response to mental tasks, allowing more blood to pool.[4]

A fast heart rate is a defining feature of POTS. An awareness of vigorous or skipped heart beats (**palpitations**) is also common. In addition, patients can experience lightheadedness, exercise intolerance, fatigue, visual blurring, weakness, imbalance, headaches, shakiness, clamminess, sweating (**diaphoresis**), anxiety, chest pain, shortness of breath (**dyspnea**), and the same type of mental fogginess those with NMH describe.[5] It is thought that the symptoms in the left column in Table 2-1 result in large part from a reduction in blood flow to the brain, and those in the right column are largely a result of the high levels of **catecholamines** (epinephrine and norepinephrine) that are part of the body's response to the reduction in brain blood flow.[6]

Symptoms of orthostatic intolerance are usually triggered in the following settings:

- with quiet upright posture (such as standing in line, standing in a shower, or even sitting still for long periods)
- after being in a warm environment (such as on hot summer days, in a hot crowded room, or in a hot shower or bath)
- immediately after exercise (during the cool-down period)

Table 2-1. Symptoms of orthostatic intolerance

Largely due to reduced cerebral blood flow	Largely due to elevated catecholamines
Lightheadedness	Dyspnea
Syncope	Chest discomfort
Diminished concentration	Palpitations
Headache	Tremulousness
Blurred vision	Anxiety
Fatigue	Diaphoresis
Exercise intolerance	Nausea

- after emotionally stressful events (seeing blood or gory scenes or being scared or anxious)
- after eating (in some), especially high carbohydrate meals, when blood shifts to the intestines during digestion
- if fluid and sodium intake are inadequate
- in association with pain
- after drinking alcohol (which causes blood vessel dilation, shunting of blood to the skin, and increased urination)
- after a period of prolonged bed rest

It is thought that we would all develop NMH with sufficiently severe environmental conditions, like not taking in enough fluids or salt or being subjected to prolonged periods of upright posture or environmental heat. The reflex response that results in lowered BP simply occurs at an earlier point in some individuals. Each person's susceptibility is affected by several factors, including genetics, diet, psychological make-up, and the presence of other medical disorders including infection, inflammation, or allergy. Some people develop NMH or POTS during tilt testing but are not affected much in regular daily life, so it is important to treat the person and not the tilt table results in isolation. An individual is treated for orthostatic intolerance when there are sufficient symptoms to interfere with normal activity.

CHAPTER 3

Diagnosis and Causes

Doctor #7 finally put his finger on it. [My daughter] was in for the usual, not feeling well, unable to sleep at night or get up for school in the morning. When he suggested bloodwork (again), she flew off the table to object and promptly passed out on his floor. He took her BP with a raised eyebrow, and then when she recovered, took it laying, sitting, then standing. He told us he suspected an orthostatic disorder and referred her for the tilt-table test. That started me on a path of internet research that led us to you, and you know the rest . . .
—Kim Hankins, a parent's view

Orthostatic intolerance, particularly NMH and POTS, cannot be detected with routine resting BP or HR screening. The diagnosis of NMH can be made with a standing test that usually lasts longer than 10 minutes or with a 30–45 minute head-up tilt table test. Although a 10-minute test is sufficient to diagnose POTS, iOH, and cOH, this is usually too brief for diagnosing NMH, which more often requires a longer period of upright posture. In our studies of individuals with ME/CFS, the median time until the development of hypotension was 29 minutes, even though symptoms were present for most within the first few minutes upright.[1]

Standing Test

Two types of standing tests can be conducted. One involves active standing, which is standing without leaning against anything.[2] The other is passive standing, which involves leaning against a wall. Few studies have compared them, but both appear capable of provoking a similar range of symptoms. The following is a modification of the passive standing test introduced by Hyatt and colleagues.[3] It begins with the patient lying supine with shoes and socks removed and with an automated BP cuff set to record BP and HR at one-minute intervals. The optimal duration of supine monitoring before standing has not been determined, and in clinical practice, the number of minutes of supine posture will vary. In balancing the desire to record a representative supine heart rate with the desire to be efficient, we have chosen to keep the patient supine for five minutes. The HR and BP are measured and recorded each minute. At the four-to-five minute point supine, we record the intensity of the patient's current symptoms (on a 0–10 scale, with 0 meaning no symptoms and 10 meaning maximal symptoms).

We then instruct the patient to stand with the heels two to six inches away from a wall and the upper back leaning against it in a comfortable but motionless position (no wiggling, shifting weight, scratching, etc.) for a maximum of 10 minutes. Each minute, we record HR and BP and ask the patient about symptoms. After 10 minutes, we instruct the patient to lie supine again, while the BP, HR, and symptom intensity are measured for another two minutes.[4]

Table 3-1. Example of a chart to record a 10-minute passive standing test. Abbreviations for specific symptoms include: FTG (fatigue); HA (headache); LH (lightheadedness); COG (cognitive symptoms); HOT (hot flash); NAU (nausea); PN (pain); SW (sweating); and ACRO (acrocyanosis)

	Blood Pressure	Heart Rate	FTG	LH	COG	HA	Other
SUPINE							
1 min							
2 min							
3 min							
4 min							
5 min							
STANDING							
1 min							
2 min							
3 min							
4 min							
5 min							
6 min							
7 min							
8 min							
9 min							
10 min							
SUPINE							
1 min							
2 min							

Tilt Table Test

Many hospitals and clinics throughout the world perform tilt table testing. It allows careful measurement of the HR and BP responses to the head-up position, usually at a 70° angle, in an almost standing position. The most common reason for performing a tilt table test in the past was the evaluation of recurrent fainting, although most now believe that it is not required for the diagnosis of recurrent syncope in those with a structurally normal heart and no evidence of a heart rhythm disturbance.[5] The history, physical examination, and **electrocardiogram** (ECG) can suffice in many individuals, and treatment can be initiated without the data from a tilt table test.

Why would tilt testing help identify the problem? Many people with NMH develop adaptations to keep from fainting, such as crossing their legs, fidgeting, or sitting or lying down when they get lightheaded or tired. During the tilt table test, they must remain still and cannot call upon these natural defenses. As a result, fainting can occur for the first time during the test. Increased fatigue and malaise often occur for a few days after the test is performed, although our experience has suggested that these residual symptoms can be minimized if the individual is treated with IV saline solutions immediately upon completion.

When neither the standing test nor the tilt table test show any abnormalities, the history becomes important for identifying low orthostatic tolerance. A new technique pioneered by Dr. Linda van Campen and Dr. Frans Visser in the Netherlands utilizes **Doppler ultrasound** techniques for measuring brain blood flow.[6] By adding flow in the four arteries that bring blood to the brain (the two internal carotid and the two vertebral arteries), they can directly measure the amount of blood flow to the brain. In studies of healthy individuals, compared to their supine values, this technique identifies an average reduction of 7% in brain blood flow after 30 minutes upright. In those with ME/CFS, the overall reduction is 26%. Among the 58% of ME/CFS adults who have a normal HR and BP response to tilt testing, it drops by 24%. For the 14% with delayed orthostatic hypotension and the 28% with POTS, it drops by 28% or 29%, respectively.[7]

What Causes Orthostatic Intolerance?

The answer to this question is not well understood. We suspect orthostatic intolerance has genetic origins in many people, because it is not uncommon for us to find several affected individuals with some form of orthostatic intolerance in the same family.[8] No gene for NMH has been identified, although one rare genetic cause has been found for a small subset of those with POTS. One trait seen with increased frequency in those with orthostatic intolerance is excessive joint mobility; some patients with joint hypermobility have a hereditary connective tissue disorder known as Ehlers–Danlos syndrome.[9] The reasons for the association between orthostatic intolerance and joint hypermobility disorders are not entirely clear, but it could be that those with joint hypermobility have more stretch in their blood vessel walls.[10] As a result, in response to higher pressures within the vein during upright posture, the leg blood vessels stretch and accommodate more blood. Not everyone with joint hypermobility and increased flexibility has orthostatic intolerance, and this physical trait can be an advantage for some athletic and artistic pursuits such as gymnastics, dance, musical performance, and swimming.

Figure 3-1 illustrates the components of a common nine-point measure of joint hypermobility known as the **Beighton score**.[11] There is some disagreement about the Beighton score that defines hypermobility at different ages. In our studies, we used a cutoff score of $\geq 4/9$. Because younger children are more flexible, and joint hypermobility

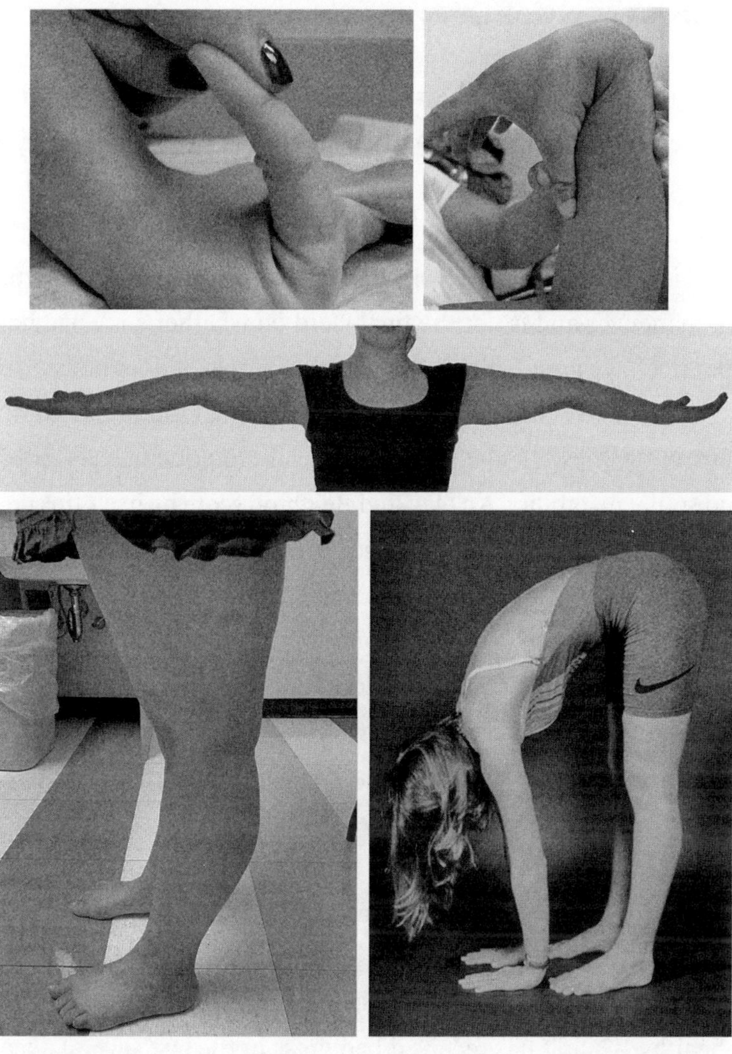

Maneuver (1 point for each positive)	L	R	Score
Passive dorsiflexion of the fifth finger at the metacarpophalangeal joint > 90 degrees			
Passive apposition of the thumb to the flexor aspect of the forearm			
Hyperextension of the elbow > 190 degrees			
Hyperextension of the knee > 190 degrees			
Forward flexion of the trunk with the knees straight so the palms rest easily on the floor			
Beighton score (≥ 4 c/w hypermobility; max score = 9)			

Figure 3-1. The elements of the Beighton score for joint hypermobility.

decreases with age, some suggest a score of ≥ 6 for prepubertal children and adolescents, ≥ 5 for those who have reached puberty and are up to age 50, and ≥ 4 for adults over 50.[12] Points are assigned as shown in the figure.

It is important to acknowledge that the Beighton score is a screening maneuver and is not the final word on whether someone has or does not have joint hypermobility. For example, it does not measure excessive laxity in the joints of the shoulders, temporomandibular joint, or the hips.[13] It also does not measure rotational hypermobility and spinal instability. An elevated Beighton score by itself (in the absence of symptoms) does not indicate a medical problem.

A number of people with orthostatic intolerance report that their symptoms began after an infection or physical trauma (such as an apparent viral illness, sinus infection, mononucleosis, Lyme disease, COVID-19, a car accident, or surgery). Some evidence suggests that autoantibodies play a role in at least a subset of patients.[14] Other environmental factors may also play a role, but more research is needed before we will know what causes either condition.[15]

One of the most common and treatable problems identified in those with orthostatic intolerance is a low salt (sodium chloride) intake in the diet. Salt helps us retain fluid in the blood vessels and maintain a healthy BP. Salt has received bad press in the last several decades because a *high* salt diet in some individuals with high or high-normal BP can lead to further increases in BP and, thereby, contribute to heart disease and stroke. This has led to general health recommendations that everyone should "cut down on salt." As we are discovering, this general recommendation is not right for all people.

In adults, an average BP is approximately 120/70–80 mm Hg. An adult's systolic BP is considered low if it is below 100 mm Hg, and it is considered high if it is above 130 mm Hg. An adult's diastolic BP is considered high if it is over 80 mm Hg. Normal values for BP in children and adolescents vary by age and weight. Individuals can have NMH at a wide range of resting BPs, but NMH is more common in those whose systolic BP is in the 90–110 mm Hg range. For individuals with orthostatic intolerance, a low salt intake can increase symptoms. In support of this idea, experimental work early in the 20th century showed that severe short-term salt restriction led to fatigue and mental dulling in the adult research participants.[16]

CHAPTER 4

Treatment

As a parent, I am feeling at a loss as to what I can do to help [my son]. I want to get him out more and moving more, but then he becomes over-tired during outings. The tiredness then carries over into the school days making school difficult. There are times when I feel he was doing better when he was not trying to get to school and was able to go to physical therapy and exercise here at home. Add to that the stress of missing so much school and constantly playing catch up.
—Rina Chios, parent of two affected children

Because patients with orthostatic intolerance have a different mix of underlying contributors, therapy must be tailored to the individual. Identifying the optimal treatment for each person can take time and requires a willingness to engage in a variety of approaches, including lifestyle changes, attention to physical therapy and activity, and medication trials. Our approach is based on the available evidence from formal studies and from our experiences treating many patients over 30 years. We use a stepped approach. Step one focuses on treatments that do not require medications (termed the *nonpharmacologic* approach), step two addresses the treatment of comorbid medical conditions, and step three involves rational and judicious use of one or more medications.

Step 1: Begin Nonpharmacological Treatments

Figure 4-1 identifies the main nonpharmacological interventions.

Avoid Prolonged Sitting, Quiet Standing, Warm Environments, and Vasodilating Medications

Where practical, avoid circumstances that commonly bring on symptoms. For example, shop at nonpeak hours to avoid long lines. Take shorter showers and baths and aim for a cooler water temperature.

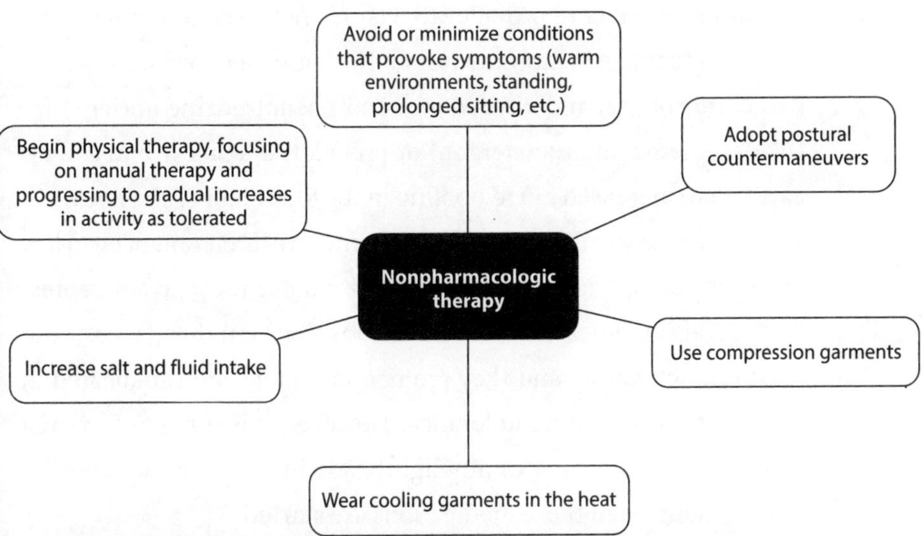

Figure 4-1. Nonpharmacologic therapy options for managing orthostatic intolerance.

Avoid saunas, hot tubs, and lying on hot beaches. Avoid sitting or standing still for prolonged periods, especially in hot weather or environments. Flex the leg muscles and shift the body weight from one leg to the other when standing still. Limit or avoid alcohol, because it causes fluid loss (through increased urination) and often leads to blood vessel dilation (commonly seen as facial flushing), which can divert blood away from the central circulation. In fact, many with orthostatic intolerance are quite sensitive to alcohol and feel sick drinking even small amounts. High carbohydrate meals have been shown to reduce blood vessel constriction in response to upright stress, so a lower carbohydrate intake and frequent small meals may help. Caffeine intake (including caffeine in soft drinks) affects some people with orthostatic intolerance positively and some in an adverse way, so examine whether caffeine is helping or making symptoms worse.

An important aspect of treating orthostatic intolerance is to review the current medications and nutritional supplements with one's doctor or health care provider to ensure that they do not have the potential to make symptoms worse. Narcotic medications (like codeine, morphine, and oxycodone) and phenothiazine antiemetics (like promethazine [Phenergan] or prochlorperazine [Compazine]) can lead to increased blood pooling in the lower half of the body. Niacin can cause vasodilation. Some patients are intolerant of even low doses of nortriptyline, amitriptyline, or similar tricyclic antidepressants. These medications can be helpful for pain, headaches, and mast cell activation, and they are not absolutely contraindicated in those with orthostatic intolerance. However, it is prudent to watch carefully for worsening of any lightheadedness or development of hypotension when these medications are started.

Use Postural Maneuvers, Compression Garments,
and Cooling Garments

Certain postures and physical maneuvers can reduce orthostatic symptoms, mainly by using leg muscle contractions to pump blood back to the heart and by compressing the abdomen to reduce the amount of blood that pools in the intestinal circulation.[1] These small changes can be important, as even a small increase in blood return to the heart can help maintain an adequate blood flow to the brain. Many patients have adopted these postures without knowing why. The maneuvers include:

- standing with legs crossed
- squatting
- standing with one leg on a chair
- bending forward from the waist (such as leaning over a shopping cart)
- sitting in the knee–chest position
- sitting with the knees higher than the hips (such as sitting in a low chair)
- leaning forward with hands on the knees when sitting
- using shoes with a higher heel to help with calf muscle contraction

Some of these postures are less conspicuous than others. Sitting in a low chair (such as a camping stool) is helpful because it brings the legs up toward the abdomen and probably reduces the amount of blood pooling in the intestinal circulation. For similar reasons, avoid sitting in a high chair with the legs dangling freely, because there is no resistance to blood pooling unless the muscles are actively contracting. One young woman found that she could sit longer without symptoms if she put her feet on a low footrest (this probably required

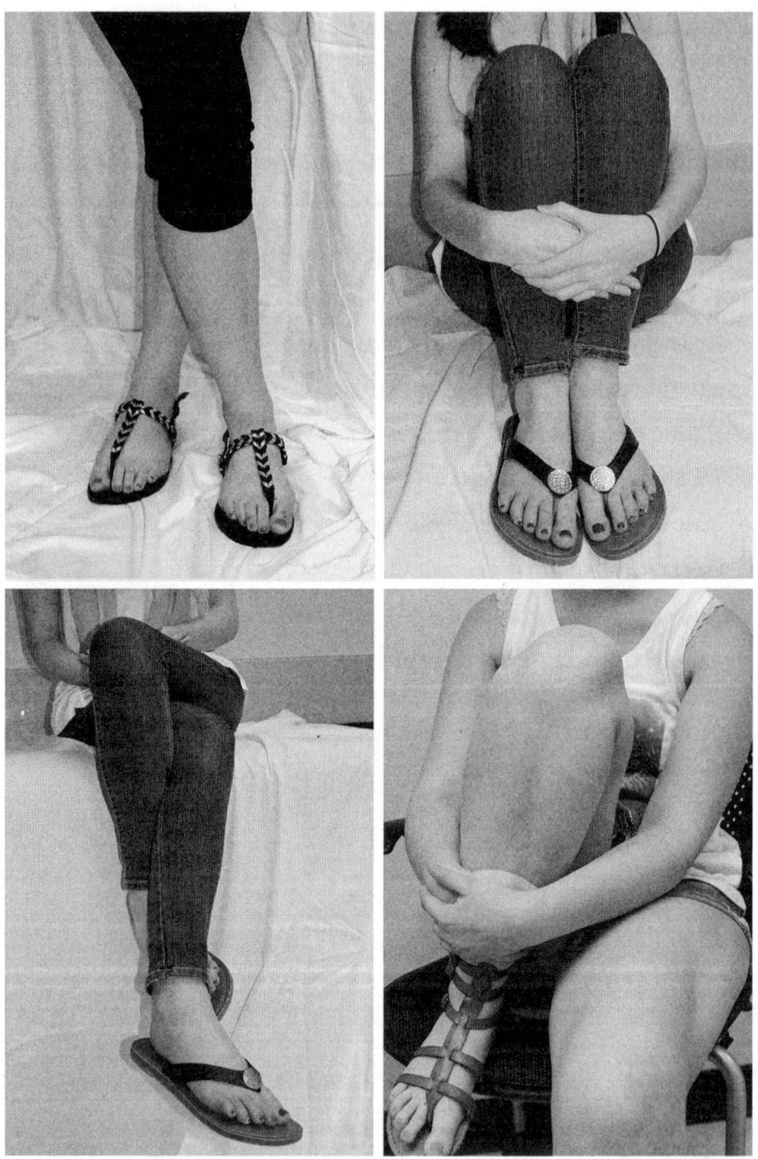

Figure 4-2. Common postures adopted by people with orthostatic intolerance.

more leg muscle contraction than regular sitting and may have also compressed the abdomen better). Some patients get worse if they adopt these postures, so they may not be right for everyone. Moving the legs around or actively clenching the fists before getting up can help as well.

Another time-honored recommendation is to elevate the head of the bed slightly by 10-15° so that the head is higher than the feet.[2] The bed frame itself must be elevated (for example, using two red bricks under each upper bed post). Using a wedge pillow to elevate the person's trunk will not have the same effect. This position helps the body retain blood volume at night. Some patients with severe ME/CFS can experience worse brain blood flow in this position, so it may not be tolerated by all.

In the research setting, several studies have shown that if blood vessels can be compressed from the outside (using tight compression garments or military antishock trousers), the abnormal HR and BP changes of orthostatic intolerance can be reduced or eliminated.[3] In day-to-day life, support hose can prevent some of the excessive blood pooling in the legs (waist-high stockings are more effective than thigh-high, which in turn are more effective than knee-high support socks). Garments that increase abdominal compression help prevent excessive amounts of blood pooling in the intestinal circulation. Examples include abdominal binders and body shaper garments. Most of our patients who wear compression stockings prefer the 20-30 mm Hg compression. Higher levels of compression, such as 30-40 mm Hg, can be difficult to get on and off, and those with joint hypermobility might find that the effort aggravates wrist and hand pain.

Cooling garments (including vests, neck wraps, and cooling beanies), are helpful when those with orthostatic intolerance are exposed to warm environments. Using a cooling vest in hot weather or upon arriving home after being out in the heat can help with a more rapid return of the heart rate to normal.

Increase Salt and Fluid Intake

Orthostatic intolerance is most often treated with a combination of increased salt and water intake. As mentioned, sodium helps hold fluid in the blood stream. The increased salt and water ensures that the blood vessels are filled better and that the heart receives an adequate amount of blood, even during upright posture. Drinking a glass of water before venturing out often helps people tolerate a given activity. We recommend a fluid intake for adolescents and adults of at least two liters per day. Our patients who drink fluids regularly throughout the day seem to do better than those who do not take this task seriously. As a result, it is important to have easy access to fluids at work or at school. Some people make the mistake of drinking a large volume of water without increasing salt intake, but without the added salt, the water they drink tends to be rapidly eliminated in the urine. The maximum fluid intake will vary for each patient. Excessive fluid intake above five liters per day can be associated with low serum sodium levels and can contribute to increased nausea.

Some individuals have **hypersomnolence** (excessive sleeping) and can sleep up to 20–22 hours per day, often in the early stages of mononucleosis or after other infections. Such prolonged sleeping periods will interfere with the ability to keep up with fluid needs. For those with excessive sleeping, we recommend that they be awakened after a maximum of 12 hours of sleep, move around as tolerated, and drink fluids. They may need to return to sleep afterward, but at least they will be better hydrated.

For those who have been on a low salt intake, we recommend an increase in the amount of salt they add to their food. Chapter 5 contains a list of high salt foods. For some mildly affected individuals, an increased intake of salt and fluids may be sufficient. Most of those with more severe orthostatic symptoms and impaired daily function will require one or more medications. Regardless of which medications are used, the increased salt and fluid intake should be continued. Some experts recommend electrolyte-containing fluids, either premixed or using electrolyte drink mixes. In some instances, buffered salt tablets can increase salt intake. Examples of common electrolyte drink mixes and salt tablets are listed in chapter 5.

Physical Therapy, Activity, and Exercise

The goal of managing orthostatic intolerance is to enable the individual to return to a more normal activity level. Exercise can increase blood volume and is often recommended as the initial treatment of orthostatic intolerance. This might be appropriate for those with only mild forms of orthostatic intolerance, but an important concern is that too much activity early in the treatment phase can often provoke increased fatigue and other symptoms. If each attempt at increasing activity is followed by increased symptoms and several days of inactivity to recover, this cycling between pushing and crashing can hinder progress. Activity and exercise are often better tolerated after effective management of the orthostatic intolerance is in place and after treatment of areas of tightness and mechanical dysfunction in the limbs and spine. We avoid a rigid advancement of activity because of the risk of provoking postexertional malaise. Instead, we recommend a gradual increase in activity tailored to each patient and designed to avoid postexertional symptom exacerbation.

Activity does not just mean exercise. In the early phase of treatment, starting to increase activity can involve engaging in something social, such as visiting friends or going to an enjoyable event.[4] Even showering more regularly is a way of increasing activity for those who have been quite impaired, as is doing more intellectual activities, such as reading. Each person can place a different value on which activities to introduce.

When individuals and their physicians feel it is an appropriate time to increase physical exercise, it is important to find something that does not provoke lightheadedness and to perform that activity for brief periods at first, increasing gradually. For example, one adolescent who had been ill for several years began functioning better after starting two medications directed at orthostatic intolerance. She first tried exercising on a treadmill, but this made her lightheaded, so she switched to a reclining exercise bike. Although she started with only two minutes a day, she increased this by small increments of 30 seconds whenever she had gone three days without provoking increased symptoms. She eventually reached 30 minutes three times a week after about three months. This allowed her to stop one of the two medications, likely because the activity had helped improve her blood volume.

Exercising while lying flat may be a way to start in the most severely impaired. Walking, water jogging (the water acts as a compressing force to counteract blood pooling in the limbs), stretching, and tai chi or yoga may be gentle ways to ease back into activities. Remember to warm up slowly before and cool down gradually after exercise. If exercising outdoors, remember that extreme heat will worsen orthostatic intolerance.

Our physical therapist colleagues in Baltimore, led by Rick Violand, PT, have helped us identify a relatively high frequency of postural asymmetries and areas of adverse mechanical tension in the nervous system as contributors to pain, lightheadedness, and fatigue in many of our patients with orthostatic intolerance.[5] These movement restrictions can be present even in those with generally increased joint flexibility. Increasing the degree of mechanical strain on a limb (for example, by performing a straight leg raise) can be associated with increased symptoms,[6] as can repetitive strain on areas that are already tight (for example, long strides in someone with restricted straight leg raise). The presence of such mechanical barriers to normal range of movement throughout the body has helped explain why some patients were finding that increased activity led to substantial worsening of symptoms. Among those with the worst of these postural restrictions, several weeks of gentle manual physical therapy can prepare them to tolerate the mild aerobic activity that would have caused a flare-up beforehand. We think careful attention must be paid to postural asymmetries and mobility restrictions during the physical examination. The diagnostic expertise of a physical therapist may be essential to correctly identifying these problems. Manual techniques that our colleagues often employ include gentle **neural mobilization** (or neural tension work), **myofascial release, strain–counterstrain maneuvers,** and **craniosacral therapy.** Once exercise is tolerated, building up leg strength using resistance exercises has been helpful in combating orthostatic symptoms.

Be aware that some physicians focus almost entirely on graded increases in exercise as a necessary part of the early treatment plan for all patients. As with other recommendations in this field, there is limited data on the efficacy of exercise as an effective treatment. A common approach among some physicians who are skeptical about the seriousness of orthostatic intolerance is to withhold pharmacological therapy until patients have demonstrated an ability to perform graded increases in exercise. Insistence on graded exercise before providing pharmacologic therapy can be unfair to patients, as we emphasize in Case 6 of chapter 7. The individual in Case 6 was physiologically unable to exercise without a marked increase in headaches and tachycardia until we began treatment with ivabradine to support her circulation. Once on this medication, she was able to rapidly advance exercise tolerance without provoking symptoms. Insisting that she successfully complete an exercise program before providing medication would have been like insisting that a person with asthma demonstrate the ability to run around a field before providing an inhaler, which any physician would consider cruel and unusual. Finding the right balance between too little and too much activity often requires a lot of trial and error.

Step 2. Treat Contributing Medical Conditions

Attending to other medical conditions is an important but underemphasized part of the comprehensive care of those with orthostatic intolerance. When these disorders are present, they can either aggravate orthostatic intolerance (e.g., by causing more lightheadedness) or their symptoms can confuse the overall picture, thereby obscuring the effects of treatments specifically directed at orthostatic intolerance. Figure 4-3 illustrates some of the common comorbid conditions we see in our patients with orthostatic intolerance, although this diagram is not meant to be exhaustive.

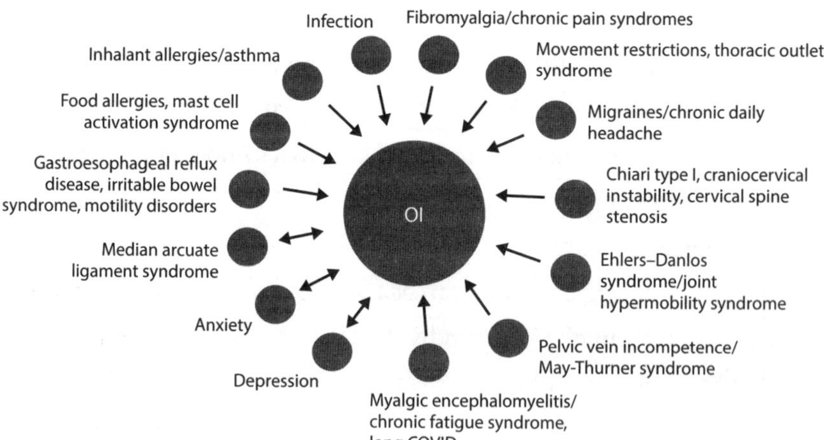

Figure 4-3. Common comorbid conditions among those with orthostatic intolerance (OI).

ME/CFS and COVID-19

As mentioned in the introduction, orthostatic intolerance is a core feature of ME/CFS. ME/CFS is diagnosed when individuals have a substantial impairment in their ability to perform previously tolerated activities, usually accompanied by profound fatigue. Other core symptoms include unrefreshing sleep and postexertional malaise, along with either cognitive dysfunction or orthostatic intolerance.[7] In our work, orthostatic intolerance is seen in over 95% of adolescents with ME/CFS,[8] and recent evidence has confirmed that 90% of adults with ME/CFS also have abnormal circulatory and brain blood flow responses to upright posture.[9] Individuals with marked impairment after COVID-19 infection (post-COVID-19 conditions, also known as *long COVID*) often have orthostatic intolerance.[10] While orthostatic intolerance is an important and treatable contributor to symptoms in both ME/CFS and long COVID, these disorders usually involve additional symptoms to those caused by orthostatic intolerance alone. For example, joint pain in ME/CFS or taste and smell disorders in long COVID are likely due to some other disease process. Treatment of the orthostatic intolerance can lead to improvement in function and can clarify which remaining problems require attention.

Depression and Anxiety

The interference orthostatic intolerance can have on normal activities, school, and work can contribute to low mood and depression. When present, depression must be treated. Fortunately, many of the modern medications for depression, such as the selective serotonin reuptake inhibitors (SSRIs; Prozac, Zoloft, and Lexapro) or the serotonin–norepinephrine reuptake inhibitors (SNRIs; Effexor and Cymbalta) can have beneficial effects on circulatory function in those with orthostatic intolerance.[11] Anxiety can worsen orthostatic intolerance, because it can be associated with higher levels of catecholamines and with reductions in carbon dioxide levels when hyperventilation occurs. Low carbon dioxide in turn causes constriction of the cerebral blood vessels, which results in even more lightheadedness. When upright, some patients with orthostatic intolerance can develop a racing heart, palpitations, chest pain, and an increased rate and depth of respiration. While these symptoms are primarily a response to inadequate brain blood flow, they can be mistaken for a primary anxiety disorder or panic attack.[12]

Median Arcuate Ligament Syndrome

Median arcuate ligament syndrome (MALS) occurs when a ligament compresses the celiac artery and surrounding nerves. It has been described in association with POTS and other forms of orthostatic intolerance.[13] MALS is recognized clinically by the presence of severe **postprandial** pain, usually accompanied by unintended weight loss. Doppler ultrasound can identify increased celiac artery flow velocity during the expiratory phase of respiration, when the ligament is at its lowest point and more likely to be compressing the celiac plexus of nerves and the celiac artery. Some patients with MALS will have an **epigastric bruit**, only present during the expiratory phase. In its most severe form, MALS usually requires surgery.

Gastrointestinal Problems

The autonomic nervous system controls the movement (motility) of food and waste products through the intestinal tract. Problems with intestinal motility are not uncommon in those with orthostatic intolerance and can include **gastroesophageal reflux, gastroparesis**/delayed gastric emptying, **irritable bowel syndrome**, and constipation.[14]

Food Allergies and Hypersensitivities

Allergies or delayed hypersensitivities to food proteins (most commonly cow's milk protein, followed by soy protein and occasionally other food proteins) can coexist with orthostatic intolerance. Delayed hypersensitivities do not cause immediate or anaphylactic allergic reactions; instead, symptoms begin two to four hours or more after ingestion. Unless intolerance of specific foods is addressed, it can obscure any improvements that might otherwise come with medications and postural changes. Dr. Kevin Kelly has identified the following symptoms that should prompt us to think further about the possibility of a food hypersensitivity: upper abdominal pain, gastroesophageal reflux, and appetite disturbances (filling up too quickly and picky eating), sometimes with recurrent **mouth ulcers**, headaches, **sinusitis**, and either constipation or diarrhea.[15] If hypersensitivity to a food protein is playing a role, substantial improvements in the gastrointestinal symptoms can result from strict exclusion of the offending food from the diet. We would emphasize that this dietary treatment is not part of the routine management of orthostatic intolerance in our clinic for all patients. It is only considered when the aforementioned symptoms are present. Given the potential dangers of unsupervised diets, patients should discuss these issues with their doctor or health care provider.

Mast Cell Activation Syndrome

Another condition that can be associated with orthostatic intolerance is mast cell activation syndrome (MCAS).[16] This condition appears to be more common among those with joint hypermobility. Affected patients often have a higher-than-normal number of allergies (sometimes including bee stings), itching, intermittent rashes and facial flushing, or intolerance of multiple foods or medications. Avoiding substances that aggravate symptoms is essential as a foundation of the treatment approach. Some patients need to avoid foods that induce

hives (e.g., shellfish, fish, eggs, nuts, chocolate, berries, tomatoes, cheese, milk, and wheat), foods that cause **mast cells** to release their contents (e.g., uncooked egg whites, shellfish, tomatoes, strawberries, chocolate, and alcohol), or foods that are high in **histamine** (e.g., fermented foods, leftovers, many fin fish, canned fish, red wine, beer, dry sausages, fermented soy products, avocado, and fermented vegetables). Careful observation of how the individual responds to each of these foods is important so that the diet does not become unnecessarily restricted. Along with avoiding triggers to MCAS, many patients will benefit from one or more of the medications that can reduce the impact of released histamine. For example, helpful medications can include H1 antihistamines like cyproheptadine, loratadine, and diphenhydramine; H2 blockers like famotidine; or tricyclic antidepressants like doxepin or nortriptyline. Other MCAS treatments (cromolyn, montelukast, zafirlukast, or quercetin) can stabilize mast cell membranes, making them less likely to release their contents.

Asthma and Environmental Allergies

Preventing activation of even mild asthma and allergies has been important in keeping our patients from developing worse symptoms. In patients with asthma, we try to reduce reliance on albuterol and other beta-agonist inhalers, because they can mimic the effect of too much epinephrine and can lead to tremulousness and worse light-headedness. Ipratropium, tiotropium, and levalbuterol (Xopenex) inhalers are often better tolerated as rescue medications in this setting. Inhaled corticosteroids can reduce the reliance on albuterol as a rescue inhaler.

Infections

Several infections are capable of triggering the onset of orthostatic intolerance. A recent example has been the SARS-CoV-2 virus that causes COVID-19, but many other infectious agents have been reported to precede the onset of POTS and other forms of orthostatic intolerance. Once orthostatic intolerance is present, any new infection can aggravate symptom control, and the infectious symptoms can last for days to weeks longer than might occur for healthy individuals.

Fibromyalgia and Chronic Pain Syndromes

Fibromyalgia is characterized by widespread pain and increased discomfort in response to levels of touch and pressure that would normally be well tolerated. The overlap with ME/CFS symptoms includes a prominent degree of fatigue along with sleep disturbances, irritable bowel syndrome, orthostatic intolerance,[17] and other problems. There is no commonly available laboratory method of distinguishing fibromyalgia from ME/CFS; in fact, they overlap substantially. Fibromyalgia is seen in 30–70% of adults with ME/CFS. It is seen less often in children and adolescents with ME/CFS. Other chronic pain syndromes can also contribute to orthostatic intolerance.

Movement Restrictions

Areas of movement restriction described earlier often respond to manual therapy. These restrictions can occur throughout the body. We now ask whether patients develop arm fatigue or numbness and tingling with the arms overhead (such as with shampooing the hair or reaching up to a high shelf) or problems with the arms extended, because these symptoms can be caused by neurogenic thoracic outlet syndrome (nTOS).[18] We have noted that lightheadedness can be aggravated when patients with nTOS raise their arms overhead. Performing a straight-leg raise has also been shown in some patients to aggravate lightheadedness. Areas of movement restriction often respond to physical therapy. Those with nTOS can benefit from injection of Botox into the scalene muscles, and occasional patients require surgery to remove part or all of the first rib.

Migraines and Headaches

Lightheadedness is a common symptom in migraine syndromes, and migraines are relatively frequent in those with orthostatic intolerance. Other patients can have chronic daily headaches, some of which are made worse by upright posture.[19] Severe headaches that are worse with upright posture and improve with recumbency can be associated with cerebrospinal fluid leaks.

Neuroanatomic Abnormalities

Some investigators have noted an overlap in fatigue symptoms and conditions in which there is too little room for the spinal cord or too much ligamentous instability in the cervical spine or base of the skull.[20] When the cervical spinal canal is narrowed, typically to a diameter of less than 10 mm, the condition is referred to as *cervical spinal stenosis*. This can be congenital (from birth) or acquired, such as when a bulging disc narrows the spinal canal or compresses the spinal cord at rest or with neck movements. Chiari malformation occurs when the lower parts of the cerebellum (the cerebellar tonsils) descend below the base of the skull and cause compression of other nerve tissues or block spinal fluid flow. Typical Chiari symptoms include headaches at the back of the head (occipital headaches), made worse by straining, coughing, or looking up. Other patients have ligamentous laxity and excessive rotational movement of the first two cervical vertebrae (atlantoaxial instability) or increased movement at the skull base (craniocervical instability). It needs to be emphasized that these conditions do not explain the presence of orthostatic intolerance in the vast majority of patients, and further studies are needed regarding the best methods to diagnose and treat these abnormalities. We think of neuroanatomic causes in patients who are refractory to usual medical management, have symptoms that worsen with neck movements, and feel that their head is heavy and unsupported, especially if there are abnormalities on the neurologic examination.

Joint Hypermobility

Joint hypermobility (the ability to move the joint beyond the usual range of motion) is usually due to ligamentous laxity in those joints. Laxity of the ligaments or skin can be accompanied by the same kind of connective tissue composition in the blood vessel walls. When the individual is upright, pressure within the leg veins is higher. This increases the diameter of the vessel, which in turn causes increased orthostatic blood pooling. High rates of orthostatic intolerance are seen in those with joint hypermobility, which can occur across a spectrum of severity.[21] At the more extreme end of the hypermobility spectrum are varying forms of Ehlers–Danlos syndrome (EDS), a disorder characterized by ligament and skin laxity that can involve multisystem, widespread symptoms that include fatigue, pain, and delayed wound healing. The most common form of EDS is the hypermobile type. Those with EDS have higher rates of comorbid conditions (e.g., temporomandibular joint dysfunction, spontaneous spinal fluid leaks, and others).[22]

Endometriosis and Pelvic Pain

Endometriosis and other painful conditions can aggravate symptoms. Some people with chronic pelvic pain will have venous abnormalities including compression of the left common iliac vein (May–Thurner syndrome) or painful varicose ovarian and internal iliac veins that contribute to pelvic congestion syndrome.[23] Common symptoms of these venous abnormalities include chronic pelvic pain that worsens with standing duration, low back pain, urinary urgency, and, for women, pain with tampon insertion or intercourse. Those with May–Thurner syndrome can develop left leg swelling. Interventional radiology procedures to identify and treat ovarian and internal iliac vein varices or stenting of the compressed left common iliac vein can help reduce not only the specific pelvic symptoms but also orthostatic intolerance.

Step 3: Begin Medications

For those with more frequent or severe symptoms, the physical maneuvers, dietary changes, physical therapy of Step 1, and the management of other conditions in Step 2 may need to be supplemented by medications. As illustrated in Figure 4-4, most of the drugs commonly used for orthostatic intolerance help to (a) improve the ability of the vessels to constrict and return blood to the heart when standing, (b) increase the amount of salt and fluid the kidney returns to the circulation, or (c) reduce the heart rate or the release of and response to the catecholamines norepinephrine and epinephrine.

While many of the medications listed in Figure 4-4 have been used by physicians for years to treat orthostatic intolerance, few have been studied formally for these conditions. Some have been tested in patients who have fainted one or more times but are otherwise healthy, some have been tested in those with ongoing symptoms due to POTS, and some have been tested in NMH patients diagnosed with ME/CFS. This book is based upon available research and our experience with treating patients with orthostatic intolerance, most of whom came to see us because of ME/CFS. The treatments we list require persistence, commitment, and the willingness to try several drugs and combinations over an extended period. Because some of the drugs carry a risk of serious side effects such as elevated BP, elevated sodium, lowered potassium, or depression, careful monitoring is required.

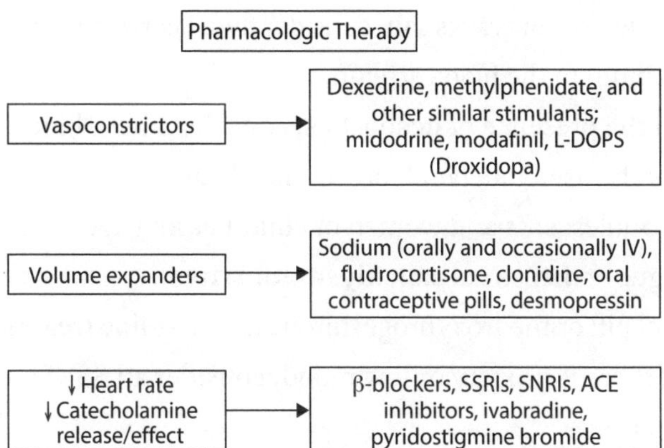

Figure 4-4. Pharmacologic therapy categories in the management of orthostatic intolerance. Abbreviations: L-DOPS (L-threo-3,4-dihydroxyphenylserine); IV (intravenous); SSRI (selective serotonin reuptake inhibitor); SNRI (serotonin norepinephrine reuptake inhibitor); and ACE (angiotensin converting enzyme).

Some of the medications no doubt work in more than one way. For example, fludrocortisone improves the ability of the blood vessels to constrict in addition to expanding blood volume. Health care providers can work with individual patients to determine the best possible combination of treatments in each situation.

Some experts recommend an algorithmic approach to the choice of medications. For example, they recommend a beta-blocker or midodrine as the first-line therapy for all patients with POTS.[24] We and others prefer an individualized approach in which medication selection is based on a variety of clinical factors, including resting HR and BP, and whether two problems can be treated with a single medication.[25] Examples of the individualized approach include the following:

- If systolic BP is relatively low for the individual's age, consider fludrocortisone or midodrine.
- If HR is relatively high at baseline, consider a beta-blocker (or ivabradine if greater than 100 bpm).

- If the patient craves salt, consider fludrocortisone to help retain sodium in the blood stream.
- In the presence of headaches, consider a beta-blocker (which can be used independently for headaches).
- If adolescents and women of child-bearing age have worse fatigue or menstrual pain (**dysmenorrhea**), consider a birth control pill or medroxyprogesterone as a first-line treatment.[26]
- If there is anxiety or low mood, consider an SSRI or an SNRI first.
- For those with suspected ligamentous laxity in whom vascular compliance might be increased, consider a vasoconstrictor (stimulant or midodrine).
- In those with prominent cognitive fogginess, consider a stimulant or clonidine.
- In those with increased nighttime urination (nocturia), consider desmopressin.
- In those with excessive sweating (**hyperhidrosis**), consider clonidine at night.

Does Treatment Cure the Problem?

It must be stressed that, when successful, the medications for orthostatic intolerance usually do not *cure* the problem. Rather, they help control symptoms and allow a more normal level of activity. After a variable period of improved function, some patients tolerate stopping medications. If it is unclear whether medicines are still working, they can be discontinued. For students, we often suggest trials of weaning a given medication at the time of a holiday or in the summer to avoid causing a downturn when school is in session.

Many with orthostatic intolerance have symptoms resurface or worsen at busy or stressful times (e.g., making an oral presentation, having company over, rushing on a hot day, and forgetting to drink), when they have an infection, or when their allergies are more active. The intravenous (IV) infusion of saline solutions has been shown in experimental settings to help reduce symptoms, and the judicious use of IV fluids periodically has a role.[27] We will administer warmed IV normal saline to help people tolerate important life events, such as longer examinations, weddings, school dances, and graduation ceremonies. For most adolescents and young adults, a two-liter infusion of normal saline over one to two hours is well tolerated due to the low blood volume at baseline. When possible, we try to avoid the insertion of indwelling catheters, because the risk of clotting and bloodstream bacterial infections increases the longer the line is in place. Carefully selected and more severely affected patients might need indwelling catheters when no other treatment is effective, but the gains in function and the risks of this practice need to be carefully balanced.

Even after successful treatment, many women with orthostatic intolerance describe a worsening of symptoms in the days around the start of a menstrual period. Some women choose to take birth control pills on a 28-day cycle or continuously (to have a period about every three months) in addition to their other medications. This is done to avoid symptoms related to hormonal changes and should be discussed with the health care provider. Many adult women who have orthostatic intolerance describe an improvement in symptoms during pregnancy and often describe pregnancy as the time when they felt "the best ever." The improvement may be due to an expansion of blood volume that occurs naturally by the end of the first trimester of pregnancy. Some studies suggest a trend toward further improvement in the second and third trimesters, possibly due to further expansion of blood volume.[28]

The natural history of orthostatic intolerance—what happens to individuals with orthostatic intolerance over the long term—has not been adequately studied. The optimal duration of medical treatment is still being worked out. Unfortunately, despite appropriate doses of the available medications, some people with orthostatic intolerance do not experience symptom improvement, and some are intolerant of the medications. This emphasizes the need for more research on this problem.

Finally, we suggest that patients take an active role in their care. If they have tachycardia, it will be helpful to their physician if they can bring in representative examples of the heart rate at rest. Alternatively, several devices are available to track heart rates (e.g., smart watches, telephone apps, and pulse oximeters). To monitor BP changes, we recommend a home BP monitor with a cuff that goes around the upper arm, not around the wrist or on the finger. HR and BP do not have to be taken routinely each day, but having this information during symptom flare-ups or after medication changes can provide helpful insights. Home monitoring does not replace visits to the physician or health care provider, but it can make those visits more productive, because this information may reflect how the patient is responding to a high salt/high fluid diet or to medications.

CHAPTER 5

High Sodium Diet

As a competitive figure skater, I was always afraid of gaining weight, so I never added salt to my foods and never ate any salty foods like chips or fries. When my personal trainer and physical therapist told me to start eating chips every day, I was shocked. He worked with so many figure skaters! Why would he recommend that? But I finally gave in, willing to try anything if it made me feel better. Eating chips every day didn't help my general day-to-day health, but it did pull me out of a bad episode. Now, my go-to way of coping with pre-syncope or a bad POTS episode when I'm out and about, unable to lie down and rest, is to eat a bag of chips and drink a bottle of water with an electrolyte packet in it. Even my friends and fiancée know to go get me a bag of chips or some super salty fries if I start feeling really bad!
—Lindsay Petracek, patient

According to a 2019 report from the US National Academies of Sciences, adolescents and adults require 1500 milligrams (mg) of sodium daily to maintain health.[1] Although health advice in the last two decades has suggested that a low sodium intake helps prevent heart disease and stroke, many individuals with orthostatic intolerance cannot tolerate this low of an intake of sodium. We believe that these individuals need much higher amounts of sodium than others in the population.

The exact amount needed is different for each individual and is often affected by one's taste for salty foods. A few individuals have been unable to tolerate an increase in sodium intake without developing increased weight gain, headache, or agitation. Sodium toxicity (salt poisoning) is not something we have seen in our patients with orthostatic intolerance. Salt poisoning is usually seen in settings where individuals are taking in high amounts of sodium without access to water (for example, infants or others who cannot walk or express thirst).

Table salt (sodium chloride) is an excellent source of sodium, with 2300 mg of sodium per teaspoon. Salt tablets are a way of getting enough sodium without dramatically changing the taste of foods. Table 5-1 shows two readily available brands.

Table 5-1. Ingredients of common forms of salt tablets

Name	Sodium (mg)	Chloride (mg)	Potassium (mg)
Thermotabs	180	287	15
SaltStick Vitassium	250	385	50

Table 5-2. Common brands of rehydration fluids

Product	Sodium (mg)	Potassium (mg)
TriOral (1/2 packet [10.3 g]/17 oz)	1300	750
Ceralyte 90 (1/2 packet [25 g]/17 oz)	1035	400
LMNT (1 packet, 6g/16 oz)	1000	200
DripDrop (1 packet, 21 g/16 oz)	670	380
Nuun (instant) (1 tablet/16 oz)	520	385
Liquid IV (1 packet, 16 g/16 oz)	500	380
Ceralyte 70 (1 packet, 10g/7 oz)	323	160
Nuun (sport) (1 tablet/16 oz)	300	150
Gatorade (1 bottle, 591 mL)	270	80

Table 5-3. Examples of foods containing a higher amount of sodium

Foods	Sodium (mg)
Breads and cereals	
Noodles, potatoes, rice from instant mixes	500
Waffles (one)	355
Wheaties (1 cup)	270
Cheerios (1 cup)	229
Saltine crackers (6)	186
Rice Krispies (1 cup)	139
Dairy products	
Parmesan cheese (1 oz)	433
Cottage cheese, lowfat (1/2 cup)	410
American cheese (1 slice)	342
Fruits and Vegetables	
Tomato sauce, canned (1 cup)	1160
Pickle, dill (1)	1090
Tomato juice (6 oz)	460
Frozen vegetables with special sauces (1/2 cup)	375
Canned vegetables (1/2 cup)	245
Meat, poultry, fish	
Sweet-n-sour chicken	1740
TV dinner	1200
Canned chili (1 cup)	1080
Lasagna	1010
Soup, canned (1 cup)	895
Fish-n-chips (1 serving)	750
Enchilada (1)	723
Hamburger (fast food)	690
Tuna, canned (1 can)	648
Hot dog	550
Corn beef (1 oz)	530
Fried chicken (1 serving)	530
Pizza, cheese (1 slice)	500
Luncheon meat (1 slice)	300
Bacon (4 slices)	280
Snacks, condiments	
Pretzel Stix, 1 tray (28 g)	1460
Soy sauce (1 tbsp)	870
Olives, green (4)	600
Salted nuts (1/2 cup)	420
Olives, ripe (4)	400
Fruit pie (1/8 pie serving)	355

Source: These values were taken from US Department of Agriculture, "FoodData central," https://fdc.nal.usda.gov/index.html.

When individuals decide to increase their sodium intake with these salt tablets, we suggest starting with one a day and working gradually up to two tablets, three times a day. Some patients tolerate even higher doses. By stepping up the dose slowly, individuals can determine how much is optimal within this range. Remember that if sodium increases from food are effective, salt tablets may not be necessary. Salt tablets are available without a prescription.

We recommend a fluid intake of at least two liters a day. Water is fine with an adequate dietary salt intake, but some prefer sports drinks (which have the advantage of a higher sodium content). Other commercially available rehydration fluids contain substantially more sodium than sports drinks (Table 5-2).

Table 5-3 provides examples of high sodium foods.

Common Medications

When you are driving with a GPS navigation device and go off course, it tells you to immediately reverse course by making a legal U-turn. After several tries at recommending this, the machine figures out that you are really going off in a different direction and stops providing the warning messages and leaves you to your own devices for a while. With POTS/CFS, once you stop being panicked about finding the U-turn when your child is off the normal route (of attending high school, etc.) and you realize that multiple panicked attempts at finding the medication fix (perfect U-turn) are not getting you anywhere, you relax a bit and realize this is a completely different road, and that one can make progress along it, but it isn't the recommended route.

—Dr. Celia Winchell, parent

Few of the medications listed in this chapter have been tested in formal clinical trials that enrolled individuals with orthostatic intolerance or ME/CFS. Some drugs have been tested in those who faint but are otherwise healthy between episodes, and others have been tested in brief trials that demonstrate short-term efficacy. There are few longer trials available to guide therapy. Although several medications for orthostatic intolerance are prescribed in combination, rigorous studies of combination therapy have not yet been performed. The following information is based on the available research and the clinical experience of our group and others who study orthostatic intolerance. Those who are pregnant or contemplating pregnancy should discuss all medication use with their healthcare provider.

1. FLUDROCORTISONE

Brand name: Florinef

Type of drug: a mineralocorticoid steroid

Action: Fludrocortisone helps the kidney retain sodium that would otherwise be lost in the urine. It may also help blood vessels constrict more readily in response to epinephrine and norepinephrine.[1] It helps the body avidly retain sodium consumed in the diet. It does so at the expense of losing potassium into the urine, so it is important to take in adequate amounts of potassium each day on this drug. Because it can be a challenge to ensure a consistent potassium intake, we recommend supplements when people start on fludrocortisone, even when the serum potassium level is normal, because the serum potassium does not provide a good reflection of total body stores. Potassium supplements are especially important if individuals remain on the drug for several months. A sustained-release potassium preparation (containing 8–10 mEq of potassium for every 0.1 mg of fludrocortisone) given once daily has been well tolerated by our patients for over 30 years. Supplemental potassium should be stopped in the rare event that an individual is not producing urine (usually in the setting of some form of kidney disease). Supplemental potassium should be used with caution and careful monitoring. It may not be needed in patients taking medications that interfere with the excretion of potassium by the kidneys, such as ACE inhibitor antihypertensive drugs and spironolactone, which is used in the treatment of acne and excessive facial hair (hirsutism).

In our clinical trial of fludrocortisone in adult ME/CFS patients with NMH, the drug was not effective when given by itself.[2] Several studies suggest that it is helpful in treating orthostatic intolerance in combination with an increased intake of salt and other medications (e.g., with a low dose of a beta-blocker), but no rigorous studies of combination therapy have been conducted, and no studies have been performed in adolescents. Despite the results of the clinical trial, many of our adult and adolescent patients continue to benefit from fludrocortisone.[3]

Common confusions: Cortisone and fludrocortisone differ. In contrast to cortisone or prednisone, which have strong anti-inflammatory properties, fludrocortisone has a minimal anti-inflammatory effect at the doses used in clinical practice. Unlike cortisone and prednisone, fludrocortisone has no effect on blood sugar at the usual doses used for orthostatic intolerance. Fludrocortisone is *not* a muscle building (anabolic) steroid. Patients taking fludrocortisone should be on a high salt diet.

Common side effects: To reduce the chance of fludrocortisone causing an elevated blood sodium level, patients should remain well hydrated. Some individuals complain of headache after fludrocortisone and some develop worse ME/CFS symptoms (more lightheadedness or fatigue), abdominal discomfort of a new type or severity, or new chest discomfort. These symptoms usually do not disappear over time, so if they are bothersome, the drug should be stopped. Tearfulness and depression occur in fewer than 1 in 20 patients treated with this drug, but patients need to be aware of the potential for an abrupt reduction in mood when they start on the drug. If such depressed mood occurs, fludrocortisone should be stopped immediately, after which the mood returns to normal, usually within 24 hours.

Some have found that minor side effects will disappear after a couple of weeks, and it is worth persevering with the medication if they are minor. Some develop worse acne on fludrocortisone. The tablet contains a tiny amount of lactose and milk protein, so it can cause abdominal discomfort to those who are extremely sensitive to milk protein. Special pharmacies can compound the drug without lactose or milk protein.

With high or even low doses over a long period, fludrocortisone can lead to a BP elevation, especially when other medications like oral contraceptives are added to the regimen. For this reason, we recommend that BP be monitored regularly, more so in the weeks after starting the drug or after increased doses and at least monthly once a stable dose is achieved.

Suggested doses for patients with orthostatic intolerance: Because the optimal dose can vary considerably, we suggest beginning with a low dose and increasing gradually. We recommend a week of increasing salt and fluid before starting fludrocortisone to ensure better tolerance, then beginning with half a tablet per day for a week. At that point, unless there has been a marked improvement in symptoms, most patients will need to increase to a full 0.1 mg tablet daily. A slower dosage advancement is to start with a quarter tablet per day (0.025 mg). If the quarter-tablet dose is tolerated for four to seven days, it can be increased to half for four to seven days, then to three-quarters or a full 0.1 mg tablet. By stepping up the dose gradually, individuals can better determine the optimal dose (occasional patients may only need half or three-quarters of a tablet). Some patients report that splitting the dose (half in the morning and half with the evening meal) provides a more even effect, but occasionally people have to return to a once-a-day morning dose to avoid insomnia.

Each patient's response to the drug is somewhat different, so we recommend regular monitoring while the doses are being adjusted. If there is no improvement or more bothersome side effects appear (worse fatigue, worse headaches, substantial weight gain, swelling of the ankles, and depressed mood), we recommend stopping the medication. If people continue to experience some benefit from week to week at a particular dose, it makes sense to continue that dose. If there are no adverse effects on a daily dose of 0.1 mg but no impressive therapeutic benefits have occurred after about a month, we will try increasing to a usual maximum of 0.2 mg (2 tablets) per day. Some physicians recommend higher doses, but we rarely find further increases above 0.2 mg daily to be beneficial (although occasional patients tolerate as much as 0.3 mg daily). If unsure about whether the drug is having a beneficial effect, it can be stopped for a few days to see if symptoms worsen. When fludrocortisone is only partially helping, we usually continue it but add other medications to the regimen that work by a different mechanism. For an example of the use of this medication, see Case 4 in chapter 7.

Comments: It is important to ensure adequate fluid intake. We recommend checking the serum electrolytes periodically, but the optimal frequency is not established. Because licorice root can have the same effect on BP as fludrocortisone, combining these two should be avoided. If BP increases toward the upper part of the normal BP range over time, a reduction in the fludrocortisone dose is likely indicated.

2. ATENOLOL

Brand names: Tenormin (other similar medications like propranolol, metoprolol, and nadolol may be equally effective, but our greatest experience has been with atenolol, and we will focus on that medication here).

Type of drug: a beta-adrenergic antagonist (beta-blocker)

Action: Atenolol blocks the effects of epinephrine (adrenaline) and norepinephrine (noradrenaline) and acts both to decrease the heart rate and to prevent the forceful heart contractions that can occur with orthostatic intolerance.[4]

Common side effects: Some individuals complain of headaches or increased fatigue after starting atenolol, and others have worse lightheadedness or general symptoms. If these problems arise, we usually stop the medication. Like other beta-blocker drugs, atenolol can lead to constriction of the airways in individuals with a history of asthma. If cough or wheezing develop soon after starting the drug, it may need to be stopped. For those with mild asthma, our impression has been that an inhaled steroid (e.g., budesonide or fluticasone) may allow patients to tolerate the beta-blocker without increased airway reactivity. Atenolol can also cause emotional depression in some patients. Atenolol is less likely than other beta-blocker drugs (such as propranolol [Inderal]) to lead to nightmares, confusion, and hallucinations. Atenolol and other beta-blocker drugs can interfere with the body's ability to correct low blood sugar, so the drug must be used with extreme caution (if at all) in diabetics. The activity of the drug can be decreased when it is used in conjunction with nonsteroidal anti-inflammatory drugs such as ibuprofen (Motrin). We usually recommend that beta-blockers be discontinued two to three days before surgery because they can interfere with the action of epinephrine if that drug is needed to treat an allergic reaction during surgery. Beta-blockers can lower the threshold for mast cell activation, and while not contraindicated, they should be used with caution in those with MCAS and severe allergies.

Doses: The usual starting dose of atenolol for older adolescents and adults is 12.5 mg per day. We usually increase it by 12.5 mg every three to seven days until we obtain an optimal effect or until side effects or bradycardia develop. Atenolol should be increased only with caution if the resting heart rate is below 60 bpm. For those with orthostatic intolerance, we usually aim for a maximum dose of approximately 1 mg of atenolol for every kg of body weight. For example, an individual weighing 62 kg (136 lb) would likely do well with between 50 and 62.5 mg of medication per day. Higher doses of beta-blockers can cause lightheadedness and fatigue. People are unlikely to tolerate increased doses when their resting heart rate is below 50 bpm. Further study is needed to determine whether patients would do better with one form of beta-blocker (selective beta-blocker like atenolol) versus another (nonselective beta-blocker like propranolol). For an example of the use of this medication, see Case 2 in chapter 7.

3. STIMULANTS

Brand names: Ritalin (methylphenidate), Concerta (methylphenidate hydrochloride extended-release), Dexedrine (dextroamphetamine), Adderall (amphetamine or dextroamphetamine), Vyvanse (lisdexamfetamine), and others. No studies have compared the relative efficacy of one to the others for those with orthostatic intolerance.

Action: The stimulant medications available for attention deficit disorder are effective as vasoconstrictor drugs for orthostatic intolerance.[5] By improving constriction of blood vessels in the peripheral circulation, they improve the amount of blood flow returning to the heart. While there is a theoretical concern that stimulants will increase heart rate in those with POTS, our clinical experience is that they often lead to a lower resting heart rate via the improvement in blood return to the heart. These medications may also exert their beneficial effects through actions on the central nervous system.

Doses: The maximum dose depends on the individual's weight. We begin with low doses, increasing once it is clear the patient tolerates the drug.

Dextroamphetamine: Dexedrine spansules are the sustained-release capsule form of the medication. Because the spansules usually contain no milk protein, they are among the ones we use for patients with milk protein intolerance. The average starting dose for adolescents and adults is one 5 mg Dexedrine spansule each morning for three days. If there is no improvement by that time, we increase the dose to two 5 mg spansules in the morning (taken at the same time). After another three to four days, if there is no improvement, we increase to three (15 mg total) in the morning. The top dose is different for each person, and further increases may be needed.

Methylphenidate: The dose of methylphenidate depends on the individual's weight, but we usually try to aim for a dose of approximately 0.5 mg per kg of body weight. We begin with low doses of either the immediate-release or sustained-release form of the medication, increasing once it is clear the patient tolerates the drug. The starting dose for school-age children, as well as adolescents and adults, is 5 mg of the immediate-release form, given first thing in the morning, repeated if necessary four hours later. Unless the 5 mg once or twice daily is enough to control symptoms, we recommend increasing the dose to one of the following:

10 mg in the morning
10 mg in the morning and 5 mg four hours later
10 mg in the morning, 5 mg four hours later, and 5 mg four hours
    after the second dose

The maximum dose can be substantially higher, up to about 1 mg of drug for every kg of body weight, but a dose of as little as 5 mg per day may be sufficient. One adolescent, for example, had her best response on a regimen of 15 mg given three times a day.

As with the use of sustained-release dextroamphetamine, therapy can begin with the sustained-release form of methylphenidate, usually available in a 10 mg strength. The starting dose for adolescents and young adults is 10 mg of the methylphenidate sustained-release, given first thing in the morning. Unless the 10 mg daily is enough to control symptoms, we recommend increasing the dose every three to seven days by 10 mg (the entire dose is taken in the morning) until a beneficial effect is seen. Some individuals benefit from staggering the dose (e.g., 20 mg in the morning and 10 mg at noon). Occasional patients tolerate and benefit from doses above 40 mg daily.

Expected therapeutic effects: The short-acting forms of methylphenidate or dextroamphetamine usually start to take effect after 30–45 minutes, and the duration of effect is approximately four hours. The long-acting forms of methylphenidate usually reach a peak effect after 1–2 hours and continue to work for about 8–10 hours.

If the stimulant medications are working at a particular dose, we expect individuals to feel less lightheadedness, headache, or fatigue. There may also be improvement in the ability to concentrate and stay on task. Individuals usually know soon after taking the first few doses if the drug is having a beneficial effect at that dose. Stimulants are controlled substances in the United States, so the prescriptions have to be written more frequently, and physicians cannot ask for refills on the same prescription. For an example of the use of stimulants, see Case 3 in chapter 7.

Side effects: The main side effects of the stimulants are insomnia, appetite reduction, moodiness, increased anxiety, and occasionally abdominal pain. Some patients describe increased lightheadedness, agitation, and other bothersome symptoms. If these develop, we usually stop the drug and move on to other medication trials. Regular monitoring is needed to ensure that the resting heart rate remains in the normal range and that weight loss is not excessive. If tachycardia is excessive, the drug likely would need to be discontinued. While the potential for addiction to stimulants is often mentioned in the literature and tolerance can develop, we have not seen patients become addicted during the last 30 years of primarily prescribing long-acting stimulants in patients with orthostatic intolerance. Similarly, once an optimal dose is identified, we rarely see a loss of therapeutic effect over time.

When the stimulants are effective for managing orthostatic intolerance but cause an excessive appetite reduction or excessive insomnia, one way of treating these adverse effects is to add cyproheptadine, an older sedating antihistamine available in 4 mg pills or in a milk-free suspension in a concentration of 2 mg/5mL. Cyproheptadine can cause sedation and thereby treat insomnia, and it also can stimulate appetite. The usual starting dose for adolescents is 4 mg at night. If there is no change after two nights, increase to 6 mg, and if there is no change after another two nights, increase to 8 mg. If it is not causing too much sedation, it can be increased to 16 mg nightly. It can also be given in divided doses, with 2–6 mg in the morning and 2–6 mg at night, although most people manage best with just the nighttime dose. The main adverse effect is excessive sleepiness the next morning. Some treated with cyproheptadine develop an excessive appetite increase that leads to unwanted weight gain.

Comment: We have found the stimulant medications to be particularly helpful for those with a childhood history of hyperactivity or attention deficit disorder or a family member with the disorder. Our impression is that they are also helpful for individuals with ligamentous laxity, but this has not been studied formally in trials. In younger patients, stimulants can help lower the resting heart rate, but there is less information available for older adults.

4. MIDODRINE

Brand name: ProAmatine (discontinued), generic options remain available.

Type of drug: Midodrine is classified as an alpha-1 agonist or vasoconstrictor. Unlike the stimulant medications, it does not have direct central nervous system effects.

Action: The main actions of midodrine are to cause blood vessel constriction, reducing the amount of blood that pools in the abdomen and limbs and shifting that blood volume into the central circulation and up to the brain.[6]

Side effects: The main side effects from midodrine are high BP when lying down in some patients, itching (also called pruritus), pins and needles, and urinary urgency/full bladder.

There is a product warning that the drug should not be taken if the individual intends to lie down or sleep, because this can aggravate supine hypertension, but this is primarily a problem for older adults with orthostatic hypotension. Adolescents and young adults with orthostatic intolerance should not be at risk for the same degree of supine hypertension as those with orthostatic hypotension (whose average age is usually above 50 years). As a result, younger patients do not usually need to heed the package insert warning to avoid lying down or napping after taking midodrine.

Common effects to be expected include a sense of tingling of the scalp and the hair on the arms and neck standing on end. These changes are signs that midodrine is working and are not reasons to discontinue the drug.

Dose: A conservative starting dose for midodrine is 2.5 mg three times daily to ensure that the drug is tolerated. The first dose should be taken upon awakening in the morning, a second dose four hours later, and a third dose four hours after that (e.g., 8 a.m., 12 p.m., and 4 p.m.). A reasonable dose progression follows:

- 2.5 mg three times a day for 2–7 days
- 5.0 mg three times a day for 2–7 days
- 7.5 mg three times a day for 2–7 days
- 10.0 mg three times a day

If there is substantial improvement at a lower dose, then it may be wise to stay at this dose for a longer period. It is not always necessary to march up to the 10 mg three times a day dose. The drug effect lasts only about three to four hours, so the medication may need to be spaced differently once it is having a clear beneficial effect. Occasional patients benefit from up to 15 mg per dose. For an example of the use of this medication, see Case 7 in chapter 7.

Comment: Generally, midodrine and stimulants should not be prescribed together, because the combination can lead to excessive BP elevations. We attempt to stop stimulant medications before starting midodrine, although occasional patients tolerate the combination.

5. SEROTONIN REUPTAKE INHIBITORS

Brand names: The selective serotonin reuptake inhibitors (SSRIs) commonly used for orthostatic intolerance are sertraline (Zoloft), fluoxetine (Prozac), and escitalopram (Lexapro), but others in this class of antidepressant medications are likely to work as well.[7] The related class of medications known as serotonin–norepinephrine reuptake inhibitors (SNRI) have also been helpful. The most used of these are venlafaxine (Effexor) and duloxetine (Cymbalta). Duloxetine is often helpful if patients have comorbid fibromyalgia or pain disorders, because it has been proven efficacious in randomized trials among those with fibromyalgia.[8]

Action: SSRIs inhibit the reuptake of serotonin at nerve terminals, leaving more available as a neurotransmitter. Serotonin can have a vasoconstricting effect.

Doses: The doses used to treat orthostatic intolerance are similar to those used for depression; as with the other medications, it makes sense to start at a low dose and to increase gradually (allowing two to four weeks for the medication to begin working after a dose increase).

With sertraline, for example, we usually begin with a dose of 12.5–25 mg per day, increasing to 50 mg if needed after two to four weeks, then adjusting upward depending on the response.

With escitalopram, the starting dose is 5 mg per day for two to four weeks, then increasing to 10 mg per day if needed. Further gradual increases may be warranted after another month.

With duloxetine, we usually start with 30 mg each morning for two to four weeks, then increase to 60 mg per day if needed. Further gradual increases to a maximum dose of 120 mg daily might be warranted.

Side effects: Some patients describe worse orthostatic intolerance (lightheadedness or fainting) or worse fatigue on the SSRIs and SNRIs.[9] If these symptoms occur, we usually stop the drug. Other side effects can include increased bruising, sweating, weight gain, reduced libido, diarrhea or nausea, or insomnia. If reduced libido becomes a problem but the drug is otherwise helping, adding bupropion (Wellbutrin) can address that symptom. Duloxetine is contraindicated in those with uncontrolled narrow angle glaucoma. Duloxetine is used to treat urinary incontinence and can cause urinary hesitancy in those without incontinence. If this problem begins within two weeks of starting duloxetine, the drug may need to be stopped.

Like a number of other medications, the SSRIs and SNRIs are metabolized by the cytochrome P450 enzyme system. Several genetic mutations cause variability in the speed with which certain medications are eliminated, resulting in higher drug levels for slow metabolizers or, conversely, subtherapeutic drug levels for rapid metabolizers. Some medicines will compete with the SSRI and SNRI drugs and change the rate of drug elimination. These issues must be kept in mind when there are adverse effects with an SSRI or SNRI.

Lastly, serotonin syndrome can occur when we combine several medications that affect serotonin metabolism. This can include stimulant medications and SSRI/SNRI antidepressants, especially when the latter are administered at relatively high doses. Symptoms of serotonin syndrome include restlessness, anxiety, disorientation, sweating, elevated HR and BP, feeling hot, and tremor or muscle rigidity. **Hyperreflexia** on the neurologic examination is also common. Any of these symptoms occurring after a change in dosing warrant medical evaluation.

Comment: Because their primary use is treating anxiety or depressed mood, these medications may be especially helpful in patients with these symptoms, but one does not need to have them for the SSRIs to help with orthostatic intolerance.

An area of concern about this class of medications has related to the rare but serious risk of suicide in the first one to two weeks of administration. The evidence suggests that this risk is primarily seen in those who are severely depressed. In these individuals who have suicidal thoughts but are too apathetic and sluggish to act upon them, the SSRI medications can have an early activating effect. As a result, patients can have improved energy for the first one to two weeks after starting the medications, but this improved energy occurs before their moods improve. Until mood improves, the individual who remains suicidal then has the energy to act upon those impulses. The risk of suicide and major personality changes drops markedly after two weeks or so. Patients should be alert to the potential for unusual reactions and should stop the medication and check in with their physicians if they have concerns about these problems.

6. PYRIDOSTIGMINE BROMIDE

Brand name: Mestinon

Type of drug: acetylcholinesterase inhibitor

Action: Pyridostigmine bromide (Mestinon) has been used for decades to treat the neuromuscular condition myasthenia gravis, and it is also used to prevent damage from certain nerve gases during chemical warfare. Its mechanism of action is to interfere with the breakdown of the neurotransmitter acetylcholine, thereby making more available at nerve and muscle interfaces. Greater concentrations of acetylcholine in the autonomic nervous system would be expected to result in a lower heart rate. In several studies, pyridostigmine bromide was recognized to cause a slowing of heart rate. This response led some to postulate that it might be helpful for those with NMH, syncope, and POTS. Formal study has confirmed those hypotheses, and the drug has been shown to therapeutically benefit some people with orthostatic intolerance, mainly by increasing the amount of parasympathetic tone in the autonomic nervous system.[10]

Side effects: Pyridostigmine bromide is generally well tolerated, but the most common side effects are nervousness, muscle cramps or twitching, nausea, vomiting, diarrhea, stomach cramps, increased saliva, anxiety, and watering eyes. The physician should be notified if these are occurring, and if the side effects are more bothersome, the drug may need to be stopped. We find that muscle cramps and twitching do not resolve spontaneously, so we stop the medication if these occur. Pyridostigmine bromide is used by gastroenterologists to treat slow intestinal motility and can be helpful if constipation is a substantial problem.

The most serious side effects are skin rash, itching or hives, seizures, trouble breathing, slurred speech, confusion, or irregular heartbeat. Because pyridostigmine bromide can lower heart rate, it must be used with caution (and started at a low dose) in those with resting heart rates in the 50–60 bpm range and in those taking beta-blockers (atenolol, propranolol, metoprolol, and others). The drug can increase bronchial secretions in those with asthma, so it should be taken with caution in affected asthmatics. Magnesium supplements can occasionally cause problems when taken in conjunction with pyridostigmine bromide, so these should be stopped when pyridostigmine bromide is started.

Doses: In adolescents and adults with orthostatic intolerance, we have been following this dosage schedule, using the 60 mg pills or the 60 mg/5mL oral solution:

Day 1–3: 30 mg once daily
Day 4–7: 30 mg twice daily (e.g., 6–7 a.m. and 4 p.m.)
Day 8–10: 60 mg in the morning and 30 mg in the afternoon
Day 11 onward: 60 mg twice daily

For more severely affected patients, a more gradual increase in doses is warranted and can be accomplished using the 60 mg/5 mL form, starting at just 12 mg (1 mL) daily and increasing gradually to an optimal effect. Some patients experience improvement with lower doses of 30 mg once or twice daily. If a good response is achieved at a low dose, there is no need to increase further. Occasional patients benefit from a third dose during the day (morning, midday, and bedtime). One adolescent found that 45 mg in the morning, 30 mg at noon, and 15 mg at bedtime was ideal for her. Some patients with ME/CFS have been reported to do better on small doses of just 12–30 mg once daily. In patients who benefit from 60 mg three times daily, some will prefer a single 180 mg sustained-release capsule, although others find the 60 mg immediate-release tablets to be more effective. Cautious increases above 180 mg can be considered. For an example of the use of pyridostigmine bromide, see Case 9 in chapter 7.

Pyridostigmine bromide pills are gluten-free but contain lactose. The pyridostigmine bromide syrup is dairy-free, as are some brands of the 180 mg time-release form (Mestinon brand and generics by Alvogen and Oceanside are milk-free).

7. DESMOPRESSIN

Desmopressin acetate

Brand name: DDAVP

Action: Desmopressin acetate is a synthetic version of the naturally occurring antidiuretic hormone (ADH, also known as arginine vasopressin). ADH is produced in the posterior pituitary gland. The main physiological effect of ADH (and of desmopressin) is to help the kidney to conserve or reabsorb water that would otherwise be lost into the urine. Individuals with central diabetes insipidus who do not produce ADH make a large volume of very dilute urine—enough to be at risk for life-threatening dehydration. Desmopressin is also used to treat childhood nighttime enuresis (bedwetting) by reducing the amount of urine produced overnight.

In those with orthostatic intolerance, desmopressin works by reducing the amount of fluid lost into the urine, therefore increasing circulating blood volume. It has been shown in short-term physiological studies to improve heart rate and orthostatic symptoms in those with POTS.[11]

Side effects: At the dose we typically use for orthostatic intolerance, adverse effects are usually mild. When they occur, the more common of these include nausea, fatigue, and headache. Serious adverse effects are more likely to occur with high doses (which are not usually needed for managing orthostatic intolerance). The main concern is that the medication can cause excessive water retention, leading to lower serum sodium levels (hyponatremia) and an increased risk of mental status changes (including somnolence and confusion) and seizures. Care should be taken if there is simultaneous use of medications that can also contribute to hyponatremia, such as NSAIDs, carbamazepine, amitriptyline, narcotics, and others.

Dose: Desmopressin acetate can be used on an as-needed basis for special occasions or as a daily medication. The starting dose for most adolescents and adults is 0.05 mg (half a 0.1 mg strength tablet), taken at bedtime. After three to seven days, if there is no beneficial effect, the dose can be increased to one full tablet. The dose can be increased to a usual maximum of 0.1 mg, three times daily. To ensure that the medication is not lowering the serum sodium, serum electrolytes should be monitored periodically, especially near the start of therapy.

Comment: This medication can help those whose sleep is interrupted by awakening to urinate or drink fluids and for those with excessive thirst. Due to the potential for low serum sodium levels, the drug should be avoided in those with hyponatremia. When taking the medication, dietary sodium intake must be adequate. The tablets contain lactose. For those with an allergy or increased sensitivity to milk protein, DDAVP is available as a milk-free nasal spray.

8. CLONIDINE AND GUANFACINE

Brand names: Catapres (clonidine) and Tenex (guanfacine)

Type of drug: selective agonists of alpha-2 adrenergic receptors.

Action: Clonidine and guanfacine are antihypertensive medications that reduce sympathetic nervous system outflow from the brain. Their mechanism of action in those with orthostatic intolerance is unknown, but both can have a vasoconstricting effect, can slow heart rate because of a vagal effect, and can lead to an expansion of blood volume in a subset of those with orthostatic intolerance.[12] Both medications are also used as treatments for attention deficit disorder and have been reported to help reduce anxiety, reduce withdrawal symptoms in those who are on narcotic medications, reduce sweating,[13] and improve sleep when taken at night. There is also some evidence that they can improve stomach emptying in patients with delayed gastric motility. Although a randomized trial in adolescents with ME/CFS did not confirm a benefit from clonidine,[14] we have found that a subset of patients with ME/CFS can benefit from the drug.

Side effects: Side effects can include worse fatigue and lightheadedness (due to the antihypertensive effect) as well as dry mouth. If side effects are mild in the first week, we usually ask patients to continue the drug to see if they resolve and the therapeutic benefit becomes evident over the next few weeks. If side effects are more impressive, we suggest stopping. If people have been taking clonidine or guanfacine for a prolonged period, they need to wean off it slowly to avoid developing rebound hypertension.

Occasional patients for whom clonidine appeared helpful for several months have developed worse side effects later, consisting of hot flashes, low BP, and worse fatigue. In such instances, it is often wise to consider withdrawing clonidine gradually to see whether it is contributing to problems.

Doses:

Clonidine: The typical starting dose for older adolescents and adults is half a tablet (0.05 mg) at night for seven days, then increasing to a full 0.1 mg tablet at night. Higher doses are sometimes tolerated. An extended-release preparation is available.

Guanfacine: The starting dose is 1 mg daily for adolescents and adults and can be increased in increments of 1 mg weekly to a usual maximum dose of 4 mg daily. Higher doses can be associated with excessive lowering of blood pressure, and we usually find that a dose of 1–2 mg daily is optimal.

9. IVABRADINE

Brand name: Corlanor

Action: Ivabradine was introduced as a treatment for tachycardia in individuals with congestive heart failure. Because it can lower heart rate, it has also been used for the management of inappropriate sinus tachycardia and POTS. It has been used to reduce the frequency of syncope in those whose neurally mediated syncope is preceded by sinus tachycardia on tilt table testing.[15]

Ivabradine slows heart rate by selectively blocking the hyperpolarization-activated cyclic nucleotide-gated (HCN) channels in the sinoatrial node (the region of the heart that has pacemaker activity). These HCN channels are also known as the "funny channels."

Activation of the funny channel increases heart rate. Selectively blocking the channel can lower heart rate without having other important effects on BP and cardiac or autonomic function. One caveat is that if heart rate falls too low due to ivabradine, BP can also drop.

Side effects: Because HCN funny channels are also present in the retina, some individuals develop phosphenes, which are visual changes characterized by halos, colored bright lights, or kaleidoscopic effects. These are usually transient and only rarely are an indication for stopping the medication. Other side effects in those with orthostatic intolerance can include increased fatigue, lightheadedness, headache, and nausea.

Ivabradine is metabolized by CYP3A4, a cytochrome P450 enzyme. If CYP3A4 is inhibited by other medications, ivabradine serum levels can rise, causing excessive bradycardia. While taking ivabradine, individuals should avoid using the CYP3A4 inhibitors itraconazole, clarithromycin (Biaxin), telithromycin (Ketek), diltiazem (Cardizem), verapamil, or grapefruit juice. Individuals should avoid taking ivabradine with Paxlovid, the antiviral medication commonly used to treat COVID-19 infection. Ivabradine can prolong the QT interval of the electrocardiogram, which in turn can be associated with an increased risk of potentially dangerous heart rhythm disturbances. The risk of QT prolongation increases when patients are taking other medicines that can also increase the QT interval. Among the more common medications that can prolong the QT interval are azithromycin, erythromycin, fluconazole, doxepin, clomipramine, levofloxacin, and ondansetron. A more extensive list of medications that can prolong the QT interval can be found at www.crediblemeds.org.

Doses: The medication is available in 5 mg and 7.5 mg strengths. The 5 mg tablet is scored. A common starting dose for orthostatic intolerance is 2.5 mg once in the morning and increasing gradually depending on the individual response. Most adults with orthostatic intolerance respond to a dose of 5 mg twice daily. Higher doses (e.g., 10 mg twice daily) are sometimes tolerated.

Expected effects: Ivabradine would be expected to reduce the degree of tachycardia, palpitations, syncope, blurred vision, and fatigue. Because the drug lowers heart rate during exercise, it can help those who develop an excessive and inappropriate rise in heart rate soon after the onset of exercise. By doing so, it can help these patients expand their exercise volume. One of our young adult patients, for example, had a resting heart rate of 110–115 bpm, and it spiked to >180 bpm within one to two minutes of starting light exercise. This was associated with the onset of a migraine. Each increase in ivabradine lowered her resting heart rate and peak exercise heart rate. On a dose of 10 mg twice daily, her resting heart rate had fallen to 72 bpm, and she was tolerating 40 minutes of exercise on an elliptical machine with a peak heart rate of 130 bpm. On that dose, she no longer developed a headache with exercise. Her case is described in greater detail later in chapter 7 (Case 6).

Comment: Because ivabradine lowers heart rate, its main use is in the treatment of those with elevated resting or upright heart rates. It is contraindicated in those with a low resting heart rate (below 60 bpm before treatment). Calcium channel blockers should not be used in conjunction with ivabradine, and care should be taken to monitor heart rate carefully if ivabradine is used in conjunction with beta-blockers.

This chapter does not present an exhaustive list of all available medications. Some experts prescribe octreotide, calcium channel blockers, disopyramide, modafinil, and enalapril, and these might be appropriate in specific situations. Octreotide is expensive and requires an injection. Disopyramide interacts with a number of antibiotics to cause serious heart rhythm disturbances, decreasing enthusiasm for its use. Modafinil and armodafinil are closely related medications that act similarly to the stimulants, but they are expensive and insurance companies often limit their use to those with narcolepsy. Enalapril has been shown in at least one study to help prevent recurrent syncope, but it can elevate potassium levels and has the potential to cause hypotension.[16] Droxidopa has been approved by the US Food and Drug Administration to treat orthostatic hypotension resulting from dopamine beta hydroxylase deficiency, Parkinson's disease, multiple system atrophy, pure autonomic failure, or nondiabetic neuropathy. It can be helpful for patients with orthostatic intolerance but can be difficult to obtain from insurance companies.[17] The typical starting dose is 100 mg three times daily; higher doses might be required. The maximum dose is 600 mg three times daily. As with all of the medications we describe, careful dosing and monitoring is required.

CHAPTER 7

Illustrative Cases

I'd love to tell whoever is holding the purse strings what it was like to watch my once vibrant, energetic, creative, happy young teen downslide into an exhausted, confused, miserable person with chronic aches and pains, completely lacking any energy or motivation. How frustrating it was to drag her from doctor to doctor to have them find no cause; one even suggested she was "faking." And as frustrating as it was for me, I can only imagine what she was going through!

—Kim Hankins, a parent's view

Case 1

A 24-year-old female was concerned about her ability to stand for long periods of time during clinical rotations for physician assistant school. She used to be very active in gymnastics and dance but has more recently experienced symptoms that interfere with her daily life.

Comment: We usually have a higher suspicion of joint hypermobility in those whose main sport is gymnastics, dance, swimming, or cheerleading, because hypermobility can offer an advantage in these activities.

Symptoms at the time of consultation: Headaches that worsen with upright posture, when she is not drinking enough fluids, if she skips meals, and in warm environments and summer weather. She also experiences lightheadedness, often with brief periods where her vision goes black and her hearing becomes distant. Her hands and feet often appear purple, and she has a sensation of warmth when she is upright for long periods. She brings her knees to her chest when she is seated, studies lying down, and stays in motion, shifting her weight when she is standing.

History: Her headaches and lightheadedness have been present since early adolescence. The headaches occurred twice a week during high school. They would worsen throughout the school day but improve after a nap. They were less common during college when she was on oral contraceptive pills, but they occurred daily during the week she was taking the placebo pills. Now, she is off the contraceptive pills. She reports that her energy is good. Her mood is normal, and she has a laid-back disposition.

Comment: The worsening of headaches with upright posture and after sitting in school all day suggested they were due to orthostatic stress. Her posture of sitting with her knees to her chest was classic for those with orthostatic intolerance, as was her preference to study lying down.

Examination: She was a tall, thin woman. Her resting heart rate was in the 90–100 bpm range during the day. She had a Beighton score of

7/9, could easily evert her eyelids, could touch the tip of her tongue to her nose (this is called a positive Gorlin's sign), could touch her tongue to her elbow, and could place her leg behind her head. Her lumbar spine was lordotic. An EKG, **echocardiogram**, and lab work were normal. A 10-minute passive standing test was performed and the results (Figure 7-1) were indicative of POTS.

Comment: It is important for clinicians to observe for the provocation of typical symptoms during the standing test. The increase in respiratory rate toward the end of the test is often seen in those with orthostatic intolerance and appears to be a physiologic change that initially promotes increased return of venous blood to the heart. If the respiratory rate continues to be elevated, patients can develop a maladaptive drop in carbon dioxide pressure that aggravates orthostatic intolerance by causing constriction of brain blood vessels.

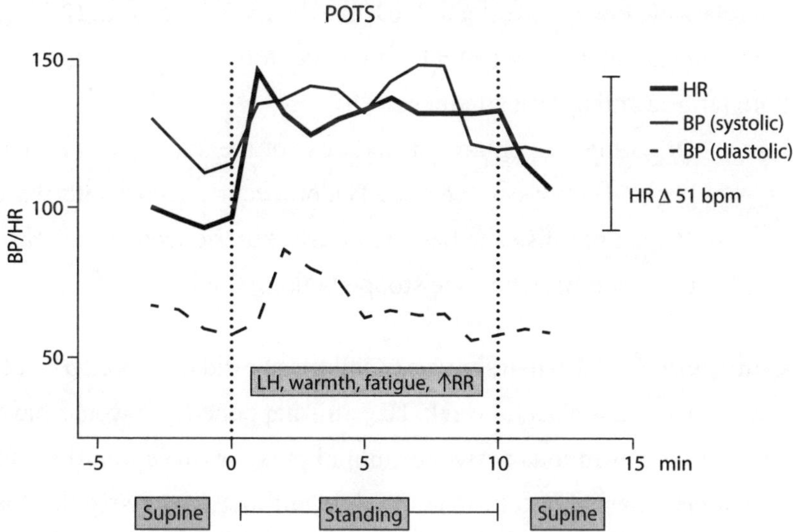

Figure 7-1. The sustained increase in heart rate from supine to standing, associated with lightheadedness (LH), warmth, fatigue, and increased respiratory rate (RR), are consistent with POTS.

Treatment:

1) We began treatment with 12.5 mg of atenolol, mainly because of her relatively elevated resting heart rate during the standing test, but also because it can be helpful for headache prevention.

She wrote the following after a month:

"The 12.5 mg of atenolol seems to be working well. My upright HR has remained lower, ranging from 60–80. Hot flashes are significantly less frequent, I have no headaches, and I'm having a much easier time exercising as well. My HR when sitting has usually been in the high 50s. I have had no side effects. BP 105/70. Do you recommend I stay at 12.5 mg or is it OK to go to 25mg?"

Comment: Given her resting heart rate in the 50–60 bpm range and the relatively low BP, we elected to leave the atenolol dose at 12.5 mg daily. Increasing the dose of a beta-blocker too much can aggravate both fatigue and lightheadedness.

2) Once she was on an optimal dose of atenolol, she resumed her oral contraceptive pills. The oral contraceptive pills were chosen because she had previously experienced an increase in symptoms when she stopped taking them.

Comment: Unlike when she was in college, she did not develop headaches during the placebo week. Had this happened, we would have prescribed continuous active hormonal pills for three months and then a brief period of four to seven days without an active pill. This continuous active pill 90-day regimen reduces by two-thirds the increases in symptoms that would otherwise occur during the week of placebo tablets in patients having monthly periods.

3) As the weather became warmer during the spring, she experienced an increase in lightheadedness and headaches. We then added midodrine to her medication regimen, starting at 2.5 mg every four hours for four doses (7 a.m., 11 a.m., 3 p.m., and 7 p.m.) and increasing gradually to 10 mg per dose. This was associated with an increase in energy and a decrease in lightheadedness and headaches.

Comment: While medications other than midodrine might warrant consideration, we started a vasoconstrictor medication with the thought that the connective tissue laxity in her ligaments was also in the blood vessel wall, and that midodrine would counteract any excessive vascular dilation in response to upright posture.

4) We explored whether dextroamphetamine (Dexedrine) might be more effective as a vasoconstrictor than midodrine, because her sister with POTS had responded well to it. On the combination of Dexedrine, birth control pills, and atenolol, she felt as well as she could imagine feeling, until she began experiencing appetite suppression, a common stimulant side effect. She was quite thin, so she had little room to lose further weight. The compromise solution was that she would take Dexedrine only on days where she was upright for longer periods and would use midodrine instead on the other days.

Ten-year follow-up: Over time, midodrine was contributing to withdrawal headaches and was stopped. She has had fewer POTS symptoms, but these continue to be more common in the heat. She eventually stopped Dexedrine because of its effect on weight loss but has continued the beta-blockers. She is off birth control, is now married, and is trying to start a family.

Case 2

A 17-year-old female presented to the clinic with fatigue, lightheadedness, and syncope, all of which limited her ability to participate in sports and social activities. The syncope had occurred more than 35 times in the preceding 18 months.

History: She was energetic and active until five years earlier, when she developed mononucleosis. She has been tired ever since. Her syncope always occurred when she was upright, never when supine or exercising. She would be groggy for several hours afterward.

Comment: Several hours of fatigue after loss of consciousness is frequently seen after neurally mediated or vasovagal syncope and helps differentiate this problem from syncope due to heart rhythm abnormalities.[1]

Examination: She had a full-body tan with no tan lines, but her physical examination, including a cardiac and neurologic examination, was otherwise normal. She did not have signs of joint hypermobility.

Table 7-1. Symptoms at the time of consultation

Symptom	Frequency	Aggravating Factors
Fatigue	Daily	Exertion, standing in line, shopping, hot days, after a bath
Unrefreshing sleep	Daily	
Lightheadedness	When she stands too quickly	Hot days, after a bath
Headaches (frontal and occipital)	Almost daily	
Syncope	>35 times in the past 18 months	

When asked to perform a 10-minute passive standing test, she was unable to stand for more than one minute before fainting, at which time her heart rate had fallen to 48 bpm (bradycardia). Blood work showed a normal complete blood count (CBC), chemistries, vitamin B12, ferritin, cortisol, aldosterone, and celiac disease screening tests. She had previously undergone an ECG, echocardiogram, 24-hour Holter study, and an exercise stress test, thereby excluding structural heart disease and making a heart rhythm disturbance less likely. A tilt table test was unnecessary given her classic history for neurally mediated syncope and absence of structural heart disease, but it had been prearranged. It confirmed the diagnosis of NMH.

Comment: A full-body tan, or bronzing of the skin, can be a physical sign of Addison's disease, an autoimmune disease of the adrenal glands. Other features of Addison's disease would usually include a low sodium level, elevation in the potassium level, and an orthostatic drop in BP.[2] This girl's full-body tan was due to her use of a tanning bed without clothing.

Treatment:

1) Treatment began with an increased salt and fluid intake. A number of medications can be helpful for treatment of recurrent syncope. We elected to begin a 0.1 mg daily trial of fludrocortisone, because this had been effective in similar circumstances in our early clinical research. Had she had even a modest improvement with the drug, we might have chosen to increase the dose. Fludrocortisone, however, had no effect on her symptoms, so we elected to stop it after one month.

2) Because fludrocortisone was ineffective, we next tried atenolol as another medication that is effective for recurrent syncope, starting with 12.5 mg daily and increasing over two

weeks to 50 mg in the morning. At a dose of 25 mg daily, she noticed improvements. We increased the dose to 50 mg daily, at which point the headaches resolved, the lightheadedness significantly decreased, and there were no further episodes of syncope. Her fatigue also improved, and she was able to resume more normal activities. Her parents and others commented on how much healthier she looked.

Comment: While it might seem counterintuitive to begin a beta-blocker in someone with syncope and a reflex lowering of heart rate, beta-blockers can prevent the initiation of the neurally mediated hypotension pathway and prevent the resulting bradycardia.[3] Beta-blockers have been used for years to prevent neurally mediated or reflex syncope. While the randomized trial evidence for effectiveness is not strong, they remain helpful for selected patients. The assumption is that atenolol blocks the effect of high circulating levels of epinephrine that are involved in the initiation of the reflex syncope pathway.

This patient had been lightheaded and fatigued for five years. Her response to atenolol illustrates the potential for a marked improvement in symptoms and quality of life when effective treatment is identified for those with orthostatic intolerance.

Case 3

A 17-year-old female was seen at the clinic for evaluation of daily fatigue and a decreased tolerance for exercise. She was able to attend school full time but had trouble concentrating and paying attention in class.

History: She began experiencing fatigue, headaches, and joint pain at age 15. She also reported painful menstrual cramps (dysmenor-

Table 7-2. Symptoms at the time of consultation

Symptom	Frequency	Aggravating Factors
Fatigue	Daily	Menstrual periods, standing in line, after exercise
Unrefreshing sleep	Daily	
Lightheadedness	Daily	
Headaches (bilateral, frontal, and occipital)	Daily	Sitting for a long time
Low back pain	Daily	Standing
Joint pain (right hip and knee)	Daily	
Right hip subluxation	Occasionally	
Lightheadedness	Common in the morning	Standing
Nasal congestion	Daily	Fall weather
Brain fog	Daily	

rhea). Oral contraceptive pills were prescribed at that time with a modest benefit. Two years later, at age 17, she developed Lyme disease that was associated with an erythema migrans rash and widespread joint pain. For this, she was treated with antibiotics for one month and experienced a resolution in the rash and widespread joint pain. Two months later, however, she developed lightheadedness, joint pain, headaches, a sore throat, poor concentration, and increased fatigue. Overall, she estimated a general wellness score of 70/100, with 100 being as good as one could imagine feeling.

Examination: Upon examination, she had nasal bogginess, a Beighton score of 5/9 (consistent with joint hypermobility), tenderness in the right hip with internal and external rotation, tenderness to palpation in the lumbar spine, and a limited range of motion on passive straight leg raise testing (this maneuver elicited stretch at just 35° of straight leg raise, which was markedly reduced for her general level of flexibility).

We performed a 10-minute passive standing test, during which she became lightheaded and had a 38-bpm increase in heart rate. Screening laboratory studies for chronic fatigue (CBC, comprehensive metabolic panel (CMP), erythrocyte sedimentation rate (ESR), thyroid hormone, iron levels, vitamin D, vitamin B12, and urinalysis) were all normal. She was diagnosed with mild ME/CFS, joint hypermobility, low orthostatic tolerance (because her change in heart rate did not meet the 40-bpm diagnostic requirement for POTS), postural dysfunctions/hip pain, dysmenorrhea and a menstrual-related increase in fatigue, and allergic rhinitis.

Treatment: We directed treatment at the various problems identified above. For her allergic rhinitis, she began an H1 antihistamine (loratadine, 10 mg daily). For the increased discomfort and fatigue at the time of her menstrual periods, we changed her to continuous active oral contraceptive pills for 84 days, then one week of placebo. We referred her to a physical therapist for evaluation of the back and hip discomfort and the range of motion restriction. For her orthostatic intolerance, we recommended an increase in salt and fluids, use of compression garments, and utilization of postural countermaneuvers.

The physical therapist identified reduced mobility in the lumbar spine along with a rotational abnormality in the pelvis. The left hemipelvis was rotated anteriorly, while the right side was rotated posteriorly. This was associated with compensatory mechanical changes in the lumbar and thoracic spine, leading to left hemidiaphragm dysfunctions that the therapist hypothesized were contributing to fatigue. The patient attended weekly sessions of physical therapy for the next three months.

At her two-month visit, her most prominent symptoms remained fatigue, lightheadedness, and problems with concentration. Stimulant medications can be effective for all three of these, and as vasoconstrictors, they may also address vessel laxity that can be present in those with hypermobility (as in Case 1). She began an extended-release form of methylphenidate initially at 10 mg each morning, increasing by 10 mg every three days as needed until she identified an optimal morning dose of 40 mg daily.

At the four-month point, her wellness score had risen from 70/100 at presentation to 82/100. She continued to improve gradually with these multimodal treatments. At the one-year follow-up visit, she reported a wellness score of 98/100. She was taking a full academic course load at her university, was walking three to four miles per day on campus, and could exercise vigorously in the gym for 45 minutes, three times a week. She required no further interventions to maintain her overall function.

Her medication delivery was interrupted for a week after the one-year point. Off methylphenidate, she immediately developed an increase in lightheadedness, headache, cognitive problems, and fatigue. These symptoms resolved when she resumed the medication.

Comment: The optimal management of orthostatic intolerance often requires effective management of other contributing conditions, in this case involving treatment of her seasonal allergies, menstrual pain and fatigue, and postural dysfunctions. The rapid return of symptoms when she did not have access to her medications illustrates two important points: 1) medications help improve function but do not necessarily cure the orthostatic intolerance, and 2) while improvement in exercise tolerance is the overall goal, our experience is that it is important to first improve the control of circulation and address movement restrictions to enable exercise without symptom exacerbation. Once activity is tolerated, it needs to be advanced in a gradual manner that avoids provoking postexertional malaise.

Case 4

A 16-year-old female was healthy and active until the gradual onset of symptoms nine months earlier. She reported fatigue, unrefreshing sleep, dizziness, headaches, and difficulty concentrating. As a result, she no longer had the physical stamina needed to attend school.

Symptoms at the time of consultation: Despite sleeping 12–14 hours per night, she had constant fatigue and would awaken unrefreshed. It was difficult to get her going in the morning. She had to lie down after showering and needed a day to recover after a relatively active day for her. She had difficulty with concentration, sore muscles, headaches, and lightheadedness.

Examination: She had prominent acrocyanosis and a Beighton score of 5/9, consistent with joint hypermobility. Her resting BP was 117/81 mm Hg. A 10-minute passive standing test was performed, during which her HR increased from 80 bpm to 121 bpm. During the standing test and a subsequent tilt table test, she reported increased fatigue, warmth, lightheadedness, nausea, and sweating. Her HR during the tilt test increased initially to above 120 bpm, followed by presyncope at 17 minutes. Her BP at that point was 78/48 mm Hg, and her HR was 70 bpm. She was diagnosed with both POTS and NMH.

Comment: If performed today, her standing test would be sufficient to diagnose orthostatic intolerance, and the tilt table test would not have been needed to initiate treatment. Her response during the tilt reminds us that POTS and NMH are not mutually exclusive diagnoses.

Treatment: Treatment consisted of an increased intake of salt and fluid, fludrocortisone (0.1 mg daily), and potassium chloride (10 mEq daily).

Within two weeks, she experienced an improvement in all symptoms. She began working two jobs, helped at her family farm, and was able to spend time with her friends again. She was able to resume school full time. Fatigue only occurred after 45 minutes of swimming. During a repeat standing test while taking fludrocortisone, her heart rate only increased 10 bpm, from 76 bpm supine to 86 bpm upright.

Ten-year follow-up: She reported a mild increase in fatigue whenever her spring and fall allergies were active. When she attempted to wean fludrocortisone in the first five years of treatment, she had a return of significant fatigue despite a good fitness level. Off fludrocortisone, she reported a wellness score of 50–70/100, whereas on the medication, her wellness score was 85–90/100. By her mid-twenties, her BP started to increase gradually, reaching 130/80 mm Hg, which was a sign that she no longer needed the fludrocortisone. She was able to wean off the fludrocortisone and potassium without any increase in symptoms.

Comment: As with Case 2, this young woman's course emphasizes the potential for marked improvement in overall function in someone meeting the criteria for ME/CFS in response to a single medication that addresses orthostatic intolerance. We are not always this fortunate, and often have to try multiple medications or combinations before a good fit is achieved.

Some authorities suggest that exercise therapy is sufficient to treat orthostatic intolerance and ME/CFS. We think this view is incorrect, and it does not accord with our experience over the last several decades. An overemphasis on exercise as the *only* treatment can be harmful to patients, especially if they develop postexertional worsening of symptoms after too much activity. Fludrocortisone was clearly supporting this patient's circulatory function and was a necessary addition that enabled her to tolerate normal activity. Even though she regained full fitness and stamina (and the same authorities would have suggested that she was thereby cured), stopping fludrocortisone was immediately followed by a resumption of her fatigue and other symptoms. This points out that improvement in exercise and activity was not sufficient to manage orthostatic intolerance in her case.

Case 5

A 15-year-old female was evaluated because she was unable to attend school. She had been healthy and active until age 12, when she developed a gastrointestinal illness that appeared to be viral. Despite improvement in her acute gastrointestinal symptoms, this illness was followed by fatigue, lightheadedness, tachycardia, cognitive problems, myalgias, and occasional headaches. She also had the emergence of generalized anxiety.

By age 15, she was only attending school part time due to her symptoms. After the 10th grade, she was unable to attend at all due to the intensity of fatigue and stamina reduction, along with lightheadedness and brain fog. A tilt table test confirmed the diagnosis of POTS, but a variety of medications, as well as those directed at her anxiety, were ineffective.

At age 19, her physical therapist appreciated increased tension in her posterior neck muscles, prompting a repeat neurologic examination, which showed an intermittently positive Hoffman sign. The Hoffman sign is a physical examination maneuver performed with a downward flicking of the middle fingertip. It is considered positive if the thumb and forefinger undergo an involuntary flexion. This physical sign is often positive in those with cervical spine abnormalities.[4] Of interest, her mother had a history of congenital cervical spinal stenosis (narrowing of the cervical spinal canal), two spinal fusions for degenerative disc disease in the neck, and two surgeries for thoracic outlet syndrome.

Examination: An abbreviated 5-minute passive standing test showed a 64-bpm increase in heart rate from supine to standing. During the test, she experienced fatigue, headache, and shortness of breath. As shown in Figure 7-2, her heart rate increase clearly met the diagnostic criteria for POTS.

To evaluate the abnormal Hoffman sign, we obtained cervical spine magnetic resonance imaging (MRI). This showed several abnormalities, including an abnormal clivo-axial angle of 117° (normal

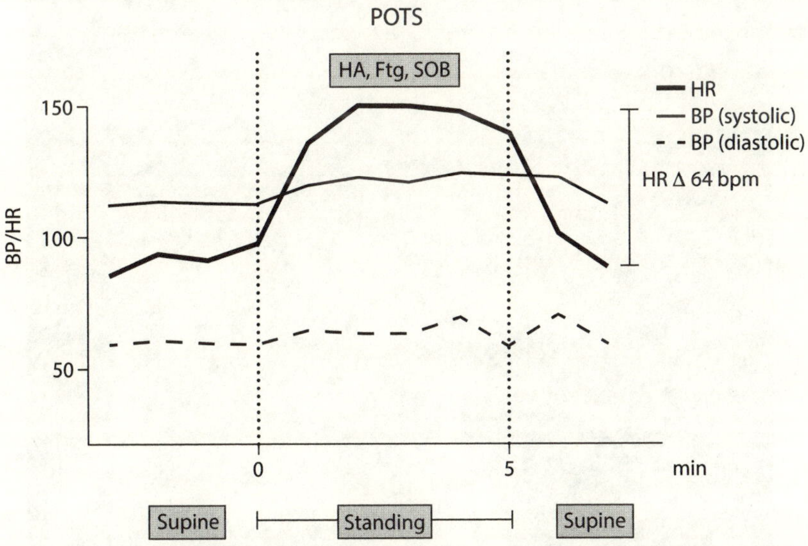

Figure 7-2. The abbreviated 5-minute standing test results in patient 5.

is 150–170°), a narrowed cervical spinal canal with an anteroposterior diameter of 8 mm (stenosis is defined as <10 mm), and a disc bulge at C6–C7 that was indenting the ventral surface of the spinal cord (Figure 7-3).

Treatment: She underwent a conservative disc replacement at the site of the C6–C7 disc bulge. Within two months, she was able to work as a dog walker and a veterinary technician. She experienced a marked reduction in anxiety, tachycardia, and lightheadedness. She was gradually able to increase her activity and exercise, including attending part-time university classes.

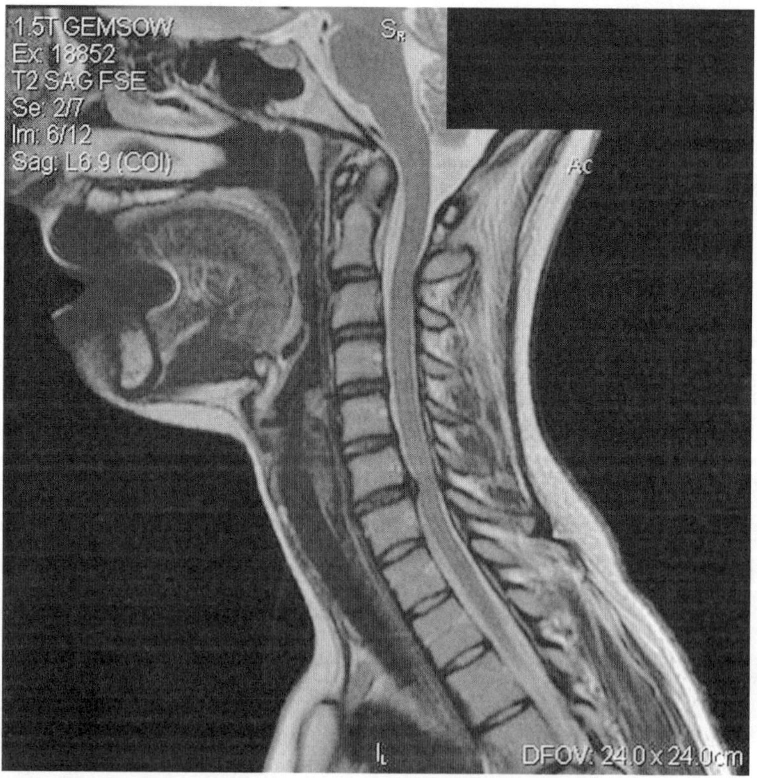

Figure 7-3. The cervical spine MRI shows a paucity of spinal fluid on either side of the cervical spinal cord, along with the disc bulge at C6–C7.

Six months after surgery, she took a summer job at a dude ranch, which involved waking up at 6 a.m., leading people on horse trail rides, and being active until late evening. At the one-year follow-up, she was a full-time college student with a part-time retail job, also working 12 hours a day on the weekends as a wedding photography assistant. Her postsurgery standing test showed a resolution of her POTS, now with only a 22-bpm change in heart rate compared to the preoperative 64-bpm change.

Comment: As this young woman's case illustrates, it is always important to ask: "Orthostatic intolerance due to what?" POTS and other forms of orthostatic intolerance can be associated with a variety of neuroanatomic abnormalities, including Chiari I malformation, cervical spinal stenosis, atlantoaxial instability, and craniocervical instability. While this patient had both an abnormal clivo-axial angle and the congenital cervical stenosis, we elected first to treat her disc bulge as the least invasive and least involved procedure.[5] This turned out to be fortuitous, because she has been fully active for the past five years and has not needed additional surgery.

Case 6

A 22-year-old came to the clinic with existing diagnoses of orthostatic intolerance, joint laxity, hypothyroidism, Raynaud's phenomenon, mild depression, migraines, and a reduced neurodynamic range of motion on physical therapy testing. She had tried numerous treatments and medications but experienced little improvement.

History: At age 14, she developed a cytomegalovirus (CMV) infection with associated fatigue, sore throat, and spleen enlargement. She had persistent fatigue afterward. She managed to complete high school and college with a full-time course load but could manage few activities other than schoolwork. She had tried many medications and treatments of her headaches and orthostatic intolerance but with no effect on symptoms. The headache treatment trials included riboflavin, coenzyme Q10, topiramate, valproic acid, pregabalin, beta-blockers, verapamil, candesartan, duloxetine, and tricyclic antidepressants. She experienced mild benefit with increased salt and fluid intake and the use of body shaper compression garments. Fludrocortisone, midodrine, stimulants, propranolol, nadolol, disopyramide, pyridostigmine bromide, clonidine, and oral contraceptive pills had no effect on her orthostatic intolerance symptoms.

After seven years of illness, her resting heart rate was 104–140 bpm with a marked increase two to three minutes after trying to exercise. Her heart rate rose rapidly to 180 bpm, and this was accompanied by a two-day exacerbation of migraines.

Treatment:

Ivabradine improved her heart rate, exercise tolerance, and cognition (Table 7-3).

Comment: This individual had inappropriate sinus tachycardia, defined as a resting heart rate exceeding 100 bpm. She had been in-

Table 7-3.   Heart rate and exercise responses to ivabradine. Abbreviations: BID (twice daily)

Ivabradine Dose	Resting HR	Exercise HR
0 mg	115	170–180 in 2 minutes with headache
2.5 mg BID	110	170–180 in 2 minutes with headache
5 mg BID	90	155, no headache
7.5 mg BID	80	140, no headache
10 mg BID	72	130, with 30–40 minutes on elliptical, no headache

tolerant of vigorous exercise due to the prompt exacerbation of migraines. Despite multiple attempts to increase her activity level, she was physically unable to without feeling worse. Ivabradine controlled her heart rate well enough that she could exercise without provoking a migraine. Her case illustrates, once again, that in many instances, people with orthostatic intolerance need medications to support their circulation before they can tolerate exercise. Even though she is now fully fit, each year she undergoes a two-week period off ivabradine while awaiting insurance reauthorization of the drug. During that time off medication, she has an immediate increase in her resting heart rate, lightheadedness, and cognitive dysfunction, all of which improve promptly upon resuming the medication.

Case 7

A 27-year-old doctoral student developed persistent fatigue, unrefreshing sleep, exercise intolerance, myalgias, and cognitive difficulties. Her medical history was notable for syncope since age 11, usually occurring twice a year, typically when standing for long periods or after a shower. She had also had frequent knee dislocations and had sustained four spontaneous pneumothoraxes (a pneumothorax is air in the pleural space between the lung and the chest wall, often caused by a weakness in the pleural connective tissue lining).

In her doctoral program, which involved prolonged sitting and listening to lectures all day, she became much more symptomatic. She experienced lightheadedness several times a day and two episodes of presyncope per week. She noted worse fatigue after her syncopal episodes. The fatigue and other symptoms interfered substantially with her attendance and overall academic performance.

She underwent a tilt table test, shown in Figure 7-4.

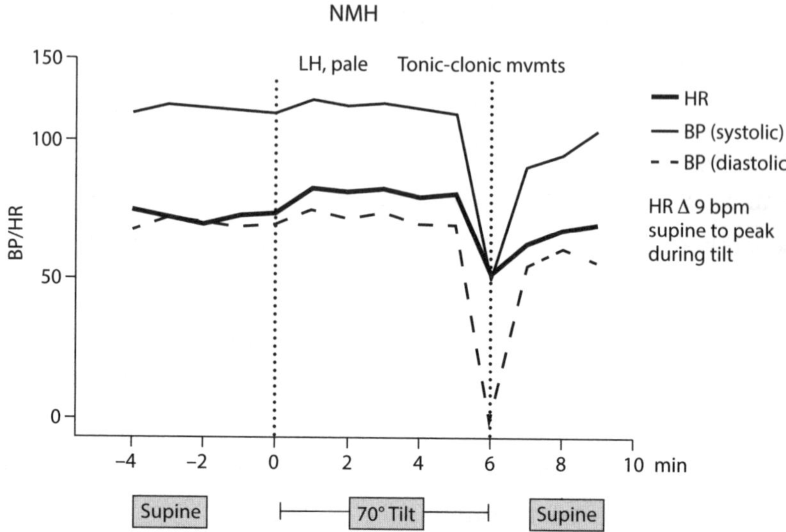

Figure 7-4. Tilt test results for patient 7. Immediately as the tilt table was brought to the 70° head-up angle, she developed lightheadedness (LH) and pallor. Her heart rate rose just 9 bpm. Her blood pressure fell abruptly at the 5-minute point, associated with a relative reduction in heart rate, consistent with neurally mediated or vasovagal syncope. Abbreviations: mvmts (movements).

A physical examination noted laxity of her joints and skin, consistent with a hereditary disorder of connective tissue. An echocardiogram excluded Marfan syndrome. Her diagnosis was Ehlers–Danlos syndrome.

Treatment: Her lightheadedness and syncope resolved with increased salt, fluids, and midodrine as a vasoconstrictor.

Comment: We selected midodrine first to overcome the increased blood pooling in the dependent circulation, which we hypothesized was caused by the laxity of her connective tissue.

She returned a year later because she was noticing persistent noncyclical pelvic heaviness and low back pain with standing. This raised concerns about her ability to tolerate standing for long periods of time, which was necessary for her occupation.

These symptoms were consistent with a condition variously termed *pelvic congestion syndrome* or *pelvic venous insufficiency*, associated with varicose ovarian veins within the pelvis.[6] This was treated with transcatheter embolization, a procedure that stopped blood flow in the dilated ovarian veins. This led to improvement in pelvic pain and further improvement in her orthostatic symptoms.

Comment: An early development of varicose veins can be associated with Ehlers–Danlos syndrome. This young woman's symptoms remind us that treatment of comorbid conditions can improve orthostatic symptoms and overall quality of life. Other vascular abnormalities that can appear and contribute to pelvic vein insufficiency include the May–Thurner anomaly, which involves compression of the left common iliac vein by the right iliac artery.[7] This interferes with optimal blood flow out of the left leg and can lead to left leg swelling and, in some instances, can create a higher risk of clot formation.

Case 8

A 16-year-old male was seen in the clinic for a three-year history of daily fatigue and lightheadedness, migraines, feeling full easily (early satiety), heartburn and gastroesophageal reflux, abdominal pain, and recurrent mouth ulcers.

History: In the first year of life, he had excessive spitting up and colic, attributed to gastroesophageal reflux. He continued to have intermittent abdominal pain thereafter, attributed to a lactose intolerance. At age 13, after a mild viral upper respiratory illness, he developed fatigue, lightheadedness, and migraines. He experienced three episodes of syncope, all while upright in a hot environment. His gastrointestinal symptoms worsened soon after the viral illness and included daily early satiety and frequent aphthous (mouth) ulcers.

He was tired on most days, worse if his sleep was interrupted. He awakened three to four times on most nights. His fatigue would worsen in hot environments. He was active in soccer and his stamina was good for one game, but he could not tolerate repeated games in a day or games on consecutive days. He had some difficulty focusing in class. His lightheadedness was occurring daily, whenever he stood up or took a hot shower. He often had to shower sitting down. He shifted his weight frequently when standing still. The migraines occurred weekly, lasting two to three days. Chronic daily headaches were also present, beginning in the morning after rising from a seated position and accompanied by dimmed vision and lightheadedness.

Examination: His physical examination was notable for two small aphthous ulcers on the inner aspect of the lower lip on the left, marked tenderness to palpation in the upper abdomen, and joint hypermobility. His Beighton score was 7/9, and he had blue sclerae, easy eyelid eversion, flat feet (pes planus), and a paper-thin, widened scar on his left knee, all features seen in those with hypermobile Ehlers-Danlos syndrome. Despite the joint hypermobility, he had several limitations in range of motion on a physical therapy examination (limited straight leg raise and limited prone knee bend). His Beck Depression Inventory score indicated a mild level of depression. He was quite symptomatic during earlier orthostatic testing by his cardiologist and had been started on fludrocortisone.

Impression: This young man had several problems contributing to his overall symptoms: migraines, orthostatic intolerance and syncope, mild depression, hypermobile Ehlers–Danlos syndrome, and areas of postural dysfunction (limited range of motion with leg movements). Based on the history of gastrointestinal symptoms and the tenderness in the epigastric area, we suspected a cow's milk protein intolerance.

Treatment:

1) We recommended a diet free of cow's milk protein. On this, his gastrointestinal symptoms resolved unless he had an inadvertent dietary re-exposure. His fludrocortisone tablet contained milk, so we had this medication compounded by a specialty pharmacy so that it contained no lactose or milk protein.

Comment: If milk, soy, or other food protein intolerance is suspected, continued ingestion of the offending food can cause persistent symptoms and interfere with interpreting the response to other interventions. In those with suspected intolerance of a specific food, we usually eliminate that food from the diet as a first step.

We often find that individuals who ultimately respond to a milk protein restricted diet had been misdiagnosed with lactose intolerance. Although one can have both lactose intolerance and milk protein intolerance, these two conditions can often be distinguished by the location of symptoms. Milk protein intolerance is characterized by upper intestinal symptoms (mouth ulcers, reflux, and upper abdominal/epigastric pain), whereas lactose intolerance symptoms are generally lower in the intestinal tract (bloating, abdominal cramping, and diarrhea).

2) At his second visit, his biggest concern was the low mood, because his upper gastrointestinal symptoms had responded

to the milk elimination. To address this, we prescribed escitalopram, starting at 5 mg and increasing after two weeks to 10 mg daily.

3) At his third visit, his mood had improved, but orthostatic migraines and some lightheadedness persisted. He also continued to have tightness on physical therapy examinations. We prescribed 5–10 mg of midodrine every four hours, three times daily (7 a.m., 11 a.m., and 3 p.m.). He also began working with a physical therapist who addressed the movement restrictions using gentle manual therapy techniques.

4) At his fourth visit, his migraines had resolved, and the range of motion of the limbs and spine had improved. He was able to gradually expand his activity level, commenting that "The more I do, the more I *can* do." A trial off escitalopram completely made his mood and headaches worse, but he was able to reduce his daily dose to 2.5 mg.

5) At the one-year follow-up, he was much improved, able to play soccer with better stamina, and able to join his high school tennis team. He had no further episodes of syncope, and only had migraines if he was not adequately hydrated.

Comment: This case illustrates the importance of addressing multiple contributors to symptoms. We suspect that treating the circulatory dysfunction with fludrocortisone and midodrine alone would not have been sufficient to bring a complete improvement. He needed to be off milk protein, needed manual physical therapy to address tightness on his physical examination, and needed to be treated for mild depression as well.

Case 9

An 18-year-old female was evaluated for fatigue, vomiting, nausea, and abdominal pain.

History: She had been an active student until age 16, when she developed fatigue during her fall cross country season, affecting her performance at competitions. The following spring, she developed strep throat, followed by a gastrointestinal illness characterized by vomiting, diarrhea, and abdominal pain for several days. Afterward, she experienced lightheadedness and fatigue as well, but vomiting and abdominal pain continued to be her most prominent symptoms.

She was diagnosed with intestinal dysmotility via an antroduodenal manometry test (a catheter that measures nerve and muscle activity in the stomach and small intestine). She also underwent tilt table testing, during which her heart rate increased by 41 bpm in the first 10 minutes (from 65 bpm to 106 bpm), without hypotension, accompanied by lightheadedness and nausea. This was consistent with POTS.

She began treatment of orthostatic intolerance with 5 mg of midodrine every four hours, three times daily and was treated with 20 mg of amitriptyline once daily for the abdominal pain and nausea. On these medications, her lightheadedness and abdominal symptoms improved, and she was able to start undergraduate courses. She had another gastrointestinal illness in April of the spring semester, with emesis (vomiting) and diarrhea for two weeks. This was associated with several absences from classes, and she subsequently took a medical leave from college. Fludrocortisone was started and increased to 0.15 mg daily but without obvious benefits.

By June of the same year, fatigue had increased to the point that she was only able to do one activity per day and spent most of the day reclining. Her wellness score at the time was 35/100. She had low mood, constant fatigue, problems with concentration, weekly headaches, and lightheadedness. Her fatigue and lightheadedness were exacerbated by activity, showers, hot environments, menses, and standing for long periods. She also had nausea most of the day, worsened by eating and by upright posture. Abdominal pain affected the entire abdomen. She experienced aphthous ulcers once a month, along with daily, frequent gastroesophageal reflux symptoms. She would drool at night (a symptom often associated with reflux). She reported constipation, for which she was taking polyethylene glycol 3350 (Miralax). She noted that milk had caused abdominal pain in the past, but she was unsure whether it was doing so at this time.

Comment: In addition to a triad of symptoms that includes epigastric pain, reflux, and early satiety, milk protein intolerance can be a cause of chronic constipation.

Other symptoms included back pain with lying down, generalized myalgias, and knee and hip discomfort before rain. She noted that she had always been an "all-purpose" worrier. Relevant family history included a brother with depression and ADHD and a mother with a milk intolerance (symptoms included gastroesophageal reflux, abdominal pain, and apthous ulcers).

Examination: At the time of the examination, her treatment consisted of an increased intake of salt and fluids, compression garments, fludrocortisone (0.15 mg daily), midodrine (5 mg every four hours, three times daily), oral contraceptive pills taken continuously for 11 weeks at a time (one menstrual period every three months), amitriptyline (20 mg daily), polyethylene glycol 3350 (17 g daily), and lansoprazole (Prevacid, 30 mg daily).

Abnormal findings included an aphthous ulcer on her lower lip and epigastric tenderness on light palpation. Her Beighton score was

2/9. She had several biomechanical abnormalities including an elevated left shoulder and a rightward tilt of the neck, along with tightness during the seated slump test and the upper limb tension test.

Treatment:

1) We diagnosed her with ME/CFS, POTS, secondary depression, movement restrictions, and suspected milk protein intolerance. The initial treatment involved having her rigidly restrict her milk protein intake, stopping fludrocortisone (which had been ineffective), optimizing her midodrine dose to 10 mg every four hours, and beginning physical therapy.

2) Off milk protein, her abdominal pain and nausea resolved. At the one-month follow-up, she had improved lightheadedness and was able to swim for 10 minutes a day. She still experienced lightheadedness daily (more if she overexerted herself). At this point, to address both mood and orthostatic symptoms, we added escitalopram (10 mg daily). Higher doses were associated with worse lightheadedness.

3) At the two-month follow-up, her wellness score was up from 35/100 to 60/100. Her heart rate would reach 170 bpm with just seven minutes of exercise on a stationary bike, confirming persistent circulatory dysregulation. A low dose of a beta-blocker caused increased lightheadedness, so it was discontinued. A trial off amitriptyline (to assess whether it was contributing to the tachycardia) was associated with worse abdominal pain, so the medication was resumed. Laboratory testing showed a low hemoglobin level of 11.4 with features of iron deficiency: a mean corpuscular volume (MCV) of 78 and a red cell distribution width (RDW) of 14.9. Supplemental iron was immediately associated with an improvement in energy and a faster exercise recovery.

4) At the three-month point, she began part-time university classes. Her heart rate would rise to 200 bpm after 10 minutes on a treadmill. She was able to attend classes for about six weeks before once again having to withdraw due to excessive fatigue. At that time, to address the POTS and the increased heart rate during exercise, we began a trial of pyridostigmine bromide and a return to more consistent physical therapy. She responded promptly to pyridostigmine and reached an optimal dose of 180 mg daily. Within a month, she was able to do more, including 45 minutes of kayaking.

5) At the seven-month follow-up, her wellness score was 75/100, she could walk for 30 minutes a day, and she was advancing in physical therapy. Compression garments helped her lightheadedness and energy, and she could go out socially more often.

6) At the eight-month follow-up, her wellness score was 85/100. She had returned to college with a reduced course load and was doing well. In addition to her daily walks, she was able to run and participate in yoga. Her anxiety and mood were improved as well.

7) At her nine-month follow-up, her wellness score remained 85/100. She could run for 20 minutes continuously on a treadmill. Her only symptoms were occasional warmth and fatigue. Her straight leg raise improved on each side from 40° to >80°. She continued her high fluid and salt intake, use of compression garments, and felt that all her medications remained necessary.

8) At the 18-month follow-up, her wellness score was 90/100, and she was able to complete a full course load in her fall semester with a 4.0 GPA and make the Dean's List. She also completed two 5K races. She experienced only intermittent

brief exacerbations in fatigue. Toward the end of four hours after taking midodrine, she noticed a slight reduction in overall function that would improve when she took her next dose.

She was able to complete a doctoral program in physical therapy, during which she remained free of fatigue or orthostatic symptoms. She was able to wean off her orthostatic intolerance medications in her late twenties, because she and her husband planned to start their family. By this point, 13 years after the onset of symptoms, she no longer required medication.

Comment: This patient required multimodal therapy, including avoidance of milk protein, a low dose of an antianxiety medication, amitriptyline for abdominal pain, physical therapy to alleviate restricted range of motion of the limbs and spine, and multiple medication trials directed at her POTS. Pyridostigmine was the most effective of her medications for POTS and was associated with the most impressive improvement in her exercise tolerance. She was diligent about gradually advancing her exercise volume, but major gains were not possible until her circulation was supported more completely with this medication.

Case 10

A 26-year-old male elite swimmer was seen for a six-month history of abnormal fatigue between workouts and an inability to practice consistently. He had also experienced headaches as an adolescent that typically improved if he laid down, and he had fainted in association with medical procedures and blood testing.

About six months beforehand, he noted that he was unable to sustain his usual swimming pace during practices, and his performance was inconsistent. During a practice that required repetitive intervals of 75 yards of freestyle swimming, he could complete the first 75 yards at an adequate pace, but the second 75 yards would be slower, and the third would be worse. He described the remainder of practice as a matter of survival.

His Beighton score was 7/9, consistent with joint hypermobility. During a 10-minute passive standing test at home, he immediately became lightheaded and nauseated. At three minutes upright, he developed arm fatigue. At six minutes, he experienced headache, and at nine minutes, he felt hot. His heart rate rose 32 bpm in association with the reproduction of his typical symptoms, satisfying the criteria for POTS. The previous fainting with blood drawing was consistent with neurally mediated (vasovagal) hypotension.

His treatment consisted of an increased dietary intake of sodium chloride, two buffered sodium chloride tablets three times daily with meals, and oral rehydration supplements. He experienced a prompt improvement in symptom severity in the first week, and by week two, he could practice consistently. To address some persistent mild lightheadedness and fatigue, in week three, we prescribed escitalopram (5 mg daily for four weeks and 10 mg daily thereafter). On this regimen, his underperformance issues resolved in practice and at national and Olympic competitions.

Comment: This case provides another perspective on the discussion of exercise as a treatment for orthostatic intolerance. Orthostatic intolerance can affect the response to performance even in highly trained athletes who could not, in any sense of the word, be considered deconditioned. In many individuals with athletic underperformance, sometimes termed *overtraining syndrome*, the medical focus has been on reducing the physical workload, looking for signs of infections like mononucleosis, and assessing for behavioral factors. A clue to the presence of orthostatic intolerance in this case was the recurrent fainting with medical procedures and blood testing along with the prominence of fatigue. We also have a high index of suspicion for orthostatic intolerance in individuals who excel at sports in which joint hypermobility is an advantage, as it seems to be in swimming.[8] Once recognized, treatment of the orthostatic intolerance was associated with a prompt return to normal training.

CHAPTER 8

Further Information and Resources

The Solve ME/CFS Initiative is an excellent source of information on ME/CFS. The website https://solvecfs.org/ lists many educational talks about aspects of the illness. Dr. Rowe's webinar presentation from September 2010 on Managing Orthostatic Intolerance is also available. It is sometimes available as a download from their website or can be found on YouTube by searching "Dr. Peter Rowe."

Other groups with helpful advice are:

The Dysautonomia International website has many helpful management ideas for patients with orthostatic intolerance and talks from conferences: http://www.dysautonomiainternational.org/

The Dysautonomia Youth Network of America: www.dynainc.org

The National Dysautonomia Research Foundation: www.ndrf.org

The Ehlers–Danlos Society: www.ehlers-danlos.com

The EDS Awareness website has many good webinars on managing aspects of disorders of connective tissue laxity: www .chronicpainpartners.com

NOTES

Introduction

1 Robinson, "Hypotension."

2 MacLean and Allen, "Orthostatic hypotension and orthostatic tachycardia";
   MacLean, Allen, and Magath, "Orthostatic tachycardia and orthostatic
   hypotension"; Chapman and Asmussen, "On the occurrence of dyspnea."

3 Shorter, *From paralysis to fatigue.*

1. Basics of Orthostatic Intolerance

1 Hall and Hall, *Guyton and Hall textbook of medical physiology*; Rowell,
   Human Cardiovascular Control.

2 Benarroch, "Physiology and pathophysiology of the autonomic nervous
   system"; Salman, "Major autonomic neuroregulatory pathways," 18.

3 Wieling and Shepherd, "Initial and delayed circulatory responses to
   orthostatic stress."

4 Vernino et al., "Postural orthostatic tachycardia syndrome (POTS)."

5 Bou-Holaigah et al., "The relationship between neurally mediated
   hypotension and the chronic fatigue syndrome"; Grubb, "Neurocardiogenic syncope."

6 Goldstein et al., "Cardiac sympathetic dysautonomia in chronic orthostatic intolerance."

7 Stewart, "Chronic orthostatic intolerance and POTS."

8 In this chapter, the definitions of orthostatic hypotension, delayed
   orthostatic hypotension, and postural tachycardia syndrome are taken
   from this consensus paper: Freeman et al., "Consensus statement on the

definition of orthostatic hypotension, neurally mediated syncope and the postural tachycardia syndrome."

9   Wieling et al., "Initial orthostatic hypotension."

10 Stewart et al., "Initial orthostatic hypotension causes (transient) postural tachycardia."

11 Adkisson and Benditt, "Pathophysiology of reflex syncope"; Benditt et al., "Catecholamine response during haemodynamically stable upright posture"; Ballantyne, Letourneau-Shesaf, and Raj, "Management of vasovagal syncope."

12 Bou-Holaigah et al., "The relationship between neurally mediated hypotension and the chronic fatigue syndrome."

13 Rosen and Cryer, "Postural tachycardia syndrome"; Schondorf and Low, "Idiopathic postural orthostatic tachycardia syndrome"; Stewart et al., "Pediatric disorders of orthostatic intolerance."

14 Grubb, "Postural tachycardia syndrome."

15 Vernino et al., "Postural orthostatic tachycardia syndrome (POTS)."

16 Brady, Low, and Shen, "Inappropriate sinus tachycardia"; Sheldon et al., "Heart Rhythm Society expert consensus statement"; Shen et al., "ACC/AHA/HRS guideline."

17 van Campen et al., "Cerebral blood flow reduced in ME/CFS during head-up tilt testing."

18 van Campen, Rowe, and Visser, "Cerebral blood flow reduced in severe ME/CFS"; van Campen, Rowe, and Visser, "Reductions in cerebral blood flow can be provoked by sitting"; Wyller et al., "Sympathetic predominance of cardiovascular regulation during mild orthostatic stress."

2. Symptoms

1   Lewis, "A lecture on vasovagal syncope"; Calkins et al., "The value of the clinical history."

2   Rowe et al., "Is neurally mediated hypotension an unrecognized cause of chronic fatigue?"; Bou-Holaigah et al., "The relationship between neurally mediated hypotension and the chronic fatigue syndrome."

3   Ross et al., "What is brain fog?"

4   Manyari et al., "Abnormal reflex venous function."

5   Low et al., "Postural tachycardia syndrome."

6   Low et al., "Postural tachycardia syndrome."

3. Diagnosis and Causes

1   Bou-Holaigah et al., "The relationship between neurally mediated hypotension and the chronic fatigue syndrome."

2   Fanciulli, Campese, and Wenning, "The Schellong test"; Streeten, Thomas, and Bell, "The roles of orthostatic hypotension, orthostatic tachycardia, and subnormal erythrocyte volume"; Plash et al., "Diagnosing postural tachycardia syndrome."

3   Hyatt, Jacobson, and Schneider, "Comparison of 70 degrees tilt, LBNP, and passive standing."

4   Roma, Marden, and Rowe, "Passive standing tests."

5   Sheldon et al., "Heart Rhythm Society expert consensus statement"; Shen et al., "ACC/AHA/HRS guideline"; Brignole et al., "ESC Guidelines."

6   van Campen, Verheugt, and Visser, "Cerebral blood flow changes during tilt table testing."

7   van Campen et al., "Cerebral blood flow reduced in ME/CFS during head-up tilt testing."

8   Camfield and Camfield, "Syncope in childhood."

9   Barron et al., "Joint hypermobility more common in children with chronic fatigue syndrome"; De Wandele et al., "Autonomic symptom burden"; Roma et al., "Postural tachycardia syndrome."

10   Rowe et al., "Orthostatic intolerance and chronic fatigue syndrome."

11   Beighton, Solomon, and Soskolne, "Articular mobility in an African population."

12   Malfait et al., "The 2017 international classification."

13   Malek, Reinhold, and Pearce, "The Beighton Score."

14   Li et al., "Autoimmune basis for postural tachycardia syndrome"; Fedorowski et al., "Antiadrenergic autoimmunity in postural tachycardia syndrome."

15   Raj et al., "Postural orthostatic tachycardia syndrome."

16   McCance, "Experimental sodium chloride deficiency."

4. Treatment

1   van Lieshout, Ten Harkel, and Wieling, "Physical manoeuvres for combating orthostatic dizziness"; Wieling, van Lieshout, and van Leeuwen, "Physical manoeuvres that reduce postural hypotension"; Smit, Hardjowijono, and Wieling, "Are portable folding chairs useful to combat orthostatic hypotension?"

2   MacLean and Allen, "Orthostatic hypotension and orthostatic tachycardia"; Ten Harkel, van Lieshout, and Wieling, "Treatment of orthostatic hypotension."

3   Rosen and Cryer, "Postural tachycardia syndrome"; Streeten, Thomas, and Bell, "The roles of orthostatic hypotension, orthostatic tachycardia, and subnormal erythrocyte volume"; Smit et al., "Use of lower abdominal

compression"; Platts et al., "Compression garments as countermeasures"; van Campen, Rowe, and Visser, "Compression stockings improve cardiac output and cerebral blood flow."

4 Rowe, "Long term follow up of young people with chronic fatigue syndrome."

5 Rowe, Fontaine, and Violand, "Neuromuscular strain"; Rowe et al., "Impaired range of motion."

6 Rowe et al., "Neuromuscular strain increases symptom intensity."

7 Institute of Medicine, *Beyond Myalgic Encephalomyelitis/Chronic Fatigue Syndrome*.

8 Roma et al., "Impaired health-related quality of life."

9 van Campen et al., "Cerebral blood flow is reduced in ME/CFS during head-up tilt testing."

10 Miglis et al., "A case report of postural tachycardia syndrome after COVID-19"; Kanjwal et al., "New-onset postural orthostatic tachycardia syndrome"; van Campen, Rowe, and Visser, "Orthostatic symptoms and reductions in cerebral blood flow"; Petracek et al., "Adolescent and young adult ME/CFS"; Dani et al., "Autonomic dysfunction in 'long COVID'"; Petracek et al., "A case study of successful application of principles of ME/CFS care"; Goldstein, "Post-COVID dysautonomias."

11 Samoil and Grubb, "Neurally mediated syncope and serotonin reuptake inhibitors."

12 Masuki et al., "Excessive heart rate response to orthostatic stress"; Raj et al., "Psychiatric profile and attention deficits."

13 Moak et al., "Median arcuate ligament syndrome"; Sandmann, Scholbach, and Verginis, "Surgical treatment of abdominal compression syndromes."

14 Sullivan et al., "Gastrointestinal symptoms."

15 Kelly et al., "Eosinophilic esophagitis attributed to gastroesophageal reflux"; Rowe et al., "Cow's milk protein intolerance."

16 Afrin et al., "Diagnosis of mast cell activation syndrome"; Shibao et al., "Hyperadrenergic postural tachycardia syndrome"; Molderings et al., "Mast cell activation disease"; Bonamichi-Santos et al., "Association of postural tachycardia syndrome and Ehlers–Danlos syndrome with mast cell activation disorders."

17 White et al., "Co-existence of chronic fatigue syndrome with fibromyalgia"; Bou-Holaigah et al., "Provocation of hypotension and pain during upright tilt table testing."

18 Jones et al., "Thoracic outlet syndrome"; Ozçakar, Ertan, and Kaymak, "Two cases and two particular signs of thoracic outlet syndrome."

19   Mack, Johnson, and Rowe, "Orthostatic intolerance and the headache patient"; Chan et al., "Intracranial hypotension and cerebrospinal fluid leak."

20   Milhorat et al., "Chiari I malformation redefined"; Prilipko et al., "Orthostatic intolerance and syncope"; Heffez et al., "Clinical evidence for cervical myelopathy"; Heffez et al., "Treatment of cervical myelopathy"; Henderson et al., "Refractory syncope and presyncope"; Henderson et al., "Craniocervical instability in patients with Ehlers–Danlos syndromes"; Rowe et al., "Improvement of severe myalgic encephalomyelitis/chronic fatigue syndrome"; Edwards et al., "Case report."

21   Rowe et al., "Orthostatic intolerance and chronic fatigue syndrome"; De Wandele et al., "Dysautonomia and its underlying mechanisms"; De Wandele et al., "Orthostatic intolerance and fatigue."

22   Castori et al., "Connective tissue, Ehlers–Danlos syndrome(s), and head and cervical pain."

23   Venbrux et al., "Pelvic congestion syndrome"; Venbrux and Lambert, "Embolization of the ovarian veins"; Knuttinen et al., "Imaging findings of pelvic venous insufficiency"; Warad et al., "Clinical outcomes of May-Thurner syndrome"; Smith et al., "Improvement in chronic pelvic pain."

24   Johnson et al., "Postural orthostatic tachycardia syndrome."

25   Bloomfield, "A common faint."

26   Boehm et al., "Neurocardiogenic syncope: response to hormonal therapy."

27   Rosen and Cryer, "Postural tachycardia syndrome"; Burklow et al., "Neurally mediated cardiac syncope"; Moak et al., "Intravenous hydration"; Ruzieh et al., "Effects of intermittent intravenous saline infusions."

28   Blitshteyn, Poya, and Bett, "Pregnancy in postural tachycardia syndrome"; Kanjwal et al., "Outcomes of pregnancy"; Kimpinski et al., "Effect of pregnancy on postural tachycardia syndrome."

5. High Sodium Diet

1   National Academies of Sciences, Engineering, and Medicine, *Dietary Reference Intakes.*

6. Common Medications

1   Chobanian et al., "Mineralocorticoid-induced hypertension."

2   Rowe et al., "Fludrocortisone acetate to treat neurally mediated hypotension."

3   Bou-Holaigah et al., "The relationship between neurally mediated hypotension and the chronic fatigue syndrome"; Fortunato et al., "Fludrocortisone

improves nausea"; Sheldon et al., "Fludrocortisone for prevention of vasovagal syncope."

4 Mahanonda et al., "Randomized double-blind, placebo-controlled trial of oral atenolol."

5 Grubb et al., "The use of methylphenidate"; Kanjwal et al., "Use of methylphenidate"; Olson, Ambrogetti, and Sutherland, "A pilot randomized controlled trial of dexamphetamine"; Blockmans et al., "Does methylphenidate reduce symptoms of chronic fatigue syndrome?"; Young, "Use of lisdexamfetamine dimesylate."

6 Ward et al., "Midodrine"; Qingyou et al., "The efficacy of midodrine"; Sheldon et al., "Midodrine for prevention of vasovagal syncope."

7 Di Girolamo et al., "Effects of proxetine hydrochloride"; Grubb et al., "Usefulness of fluoxetine hydrochloride."

8 Arnold et al., "A double-blind, multicenter trial comparing duloxetine with placebo."

9 Tandan, Giuffre, and Sheldon, "Exacerbations of neurally mediated syncope."

10 Singer et al., "Acetylcholinesterase inhibition"; Raj et al., "Acetylcholinesterase inhibition improves tachycardia"; Filler et al., "Pharmacokinetics of pyridostigmine."

11 Coffin et al., "Desmopressin acutely decreases tachycardia."

12 Robertson et al., "Clonidine raises BP in severe idiopathic orthostatic hypotension."

13 de Cássia Collaço et al., "Anxiety and dysautonomia symptoms."

14 Sulheim et al., "Disease mechanisms and clonidine treatment."

15 McDonald, Frith, and Newton, "Single centre experience of ivabradine"; Sutton et al., "Ivabradine in treatment of sinus tachycardia mediated vasovagal syncope"; Taub et al., "Randomized trial of ivabradine"; Towheed et al., "Ivabradine in children"; Annamaria et al., "Treatment of inappropriate sinus tachycardia."

16 Zeng et al., "Randomized, double-blind, placebo-controlled trial of oral enalapril."

17 Kaufmann et al., "Droxidopa for neurogenic orthostatic hypotension"; Kokorelis et al., "Successful treatment of refractory orthostatic intolerance."

7. Illustrative Cases

1 Lewis, "A lecture on vasovagal syncope"; Calkins et al., "The value of the clinical history."

2 Park, Didi, and Blair, "The diagnosis and treatment of adrenal insufficiency."

3 Grubb and Olshansky, *Syncope*.

4 Malanga, Landes, and Nadler, "Provocative tests in cervical spine examination."

5 Rowe et al., "Improvement of severe myalgic encephalomyelitis/chronic fatigue syndrome."

6 Venbrux and Lambert, "Embolization of the ovarian veins"; Smith et al., "Improvement in chronic pelvic pain."

7 Knuttinen et al., "Imaging findings of pelvic venous insufficiency."

8 Petracek et al., "Orthostatic intolerance as a potential contributor to prolonged fatigue."

GLOSSARY

Acrocyanosis A reddish-purple discoloration of the hands, legs, or feet when upright.

Beighton score A common measurement of joint hypermobility, consisting of five maneuvers and a possible score between 0 and 9, with higher scores indicating greater joint laxity.

Bradycardia Low heart rate, conventionally regarded as less than 60 bpm in adolescents and adults and less than the fifth percentile for age in younger children.

Catecholamines Neurotransmitters released in the body due to physical, cognitive, or emotional stress. The main catecholamines are dopamine, norepinephrine, and epinephrine.

cerebral blood flow The blood supply to the brain.

craniosacral therapy An osteopathic manual therapy technique that uses a gentle touch on the head, sacrum, and spinal cord to improve muscle and nerve function.

diaphoresis Sweating.

diastolic blood pressure The bottom number of a blood pressure measurement. This number is the pressure (measured in mm of Hg) in arteries between heartbeats when the heart is filling with blood.

Doppler ultrasound A noninvasive test that uses soundwaves to show the blood flow in vessels.

dysmenorrhea Menstrual pain.

dyspnea Shortness of breath; the feeling of not being able to take a deep breath.

echocardiogram An ultrasound test that checks the structure and function of the heart and its valves.

electrocardiogram A test where electrodes are placed on the chest, arms, and legs to assess the electrical activity of the heart.

endometriosis A condition in which the lining of the uterus (endometrium) is present outside of the uterus, usually associated with pelvic pain.

epigastric bruit An abnormal swishing sound heard in the upper abdomen with a stethoscope.

epinephrine A hormone and neurotransmitter. Also known as *adrenaline*.

gastroesophageal reflux When stomach contents move back up from the stomach into the esophagus. This often causes heartburn.

gastroparesis A condition in which the stomach takes too long to empty food.

histamine A compound found in cells in the body (including mast cells), important in the allergic response and capable of causing symptoms of allergic reactions such as itchiness, runny nose, redness, and sneezing.

hives Itchy welts that can appear anywhere on the body.

hyperhidrosis Excessive sweating.

hyperreflexia When deep tendon reflex responses are stronger than normal.

hypersomnolence Excessive sleepiness.

hypertension High blood pressure.

hypotension Low blood pressure.

irritable bowel syndrome A disorder affecting the intestine, causing a variety of symptoms such as abdominal pain, constipation, diarrhea, gas, and bloating.

mast cells Cells involved in host defense and allergic responses that are made in the bone marrow and migrate to tissues throughout the body, most notably the skin, airway, digestive tract, and the interface between nerves and blood vessels.

mouth ulcers Small sores in the mouth. Also known as *canker sores* or *aphthous ulcers*.

myalgias Muscle aches or pain.

myofascial release A manual therapy technique which focuses on treating tight fascia and the surrounding muscles.

neural mobilization A physical therapy technique in which light pressure and oscillatory movements are applied to nerves and their soft tissue surroundings.

norepinephrine A hormone and neurotransmitter. Also known as *noradrenaline*.

palpitations Heartbeats that are more noticeable than usual and feel like they are pounding, skipping, or racing.

phalanx Any bone of a finger or toe. The proximal phalanx is the part of the finger closest to the palm.

postexertional malaise Exacerbation of fatigue and other symptoms after physical or mental exertion, orthostatic stress, or longitudinal strain to nerves, sometimes lasting for days or weeks.

postprandial After eating.

psychosomatic A symptom or condition whose origin is psychological, not physical.

sinusitis Inflammation of a sinus, often caused by bacterial infection. Symptoms can include sinus pressure and pain.

strain–counterstrain maneuvers A technique used in physical therapy and osteopathic manual therapy, usually involving gentle mobilization of muscles and joints into positions of ease.

syncope Fainting.

systolic blood pressure The top number in a blood pressure measurement. This number is the measurement of pressure (in mm Hg) at the time the heart beats.

tachycardia High heart rate.

REFERENCES

Adkisson WO, Benditt DG. Pathophysiology of reflex syncope: a review. *J Cardiovasc Electrophysiol*. 2017;28(9):1088–1097.

Afrin LB, Ackerley MB, Bluestein LS, et al. Diagnosis of mast cell activation syndrome: a global "consensus-2." *Diagnosis (Berl)*. 2021;8(2):137–152.

Annamaria M, Lupo PP, Foresti S, et al. Treatment of inappropriate sinus tachycardia with ivabradine. *J Interv Card Electrophysiol*. 2016;46(1):47–53.

Arnold LM, Lu Y, Crofford LJ, et al. A double-blind, multicenter trial comparing duloxetine with placebo in the treatment of fibromyalgia patients with or without major depressive disorder. *Arthritis & Rheumatism*. 2004;50(9): 2974–2984.

Ballantyne BA, Letourneau-Shesaf S, Raj SR. Management of vasovagal syncope. *Auton Neurosci*. 2021;236:102904.

Barron DF, Cohen BA, Geraghty MT, Violand R, Rowe PC. Joint hypermobility is more common in children with chronic fatigue syndrome than in healthy controls. *J Pediatr*. 2002;141:421–425.

Beighton P, Solomon L, Soskolne CL. Articular mobility in an African population. *Ann Rheum Dis*. 1973;32:413–418.

Benarroch EE. Physiology and pathophysiology of the autonomic nervous system. *Continuum (Minneap Minn)*. 2020;26(1):12–24.

Benditt DG, Ermis C, Padanilam B, Samniah N, Sakaguchi S. Catecholamine response during haemodynamically stable upright posture in individuals with and without tilt-table induced vasovagal syncope. *Europace*. 2003; 5(1):65–70.

Blitshteyn S, Poya H, Bett GC. Pregnancy in postural tachycardia syndrome: clinical course and maternal and fetal outcomes. *J Matern Fetal Neonatal Med*. 2012;25(9):1631-1634.

Blockmans D, Persoons P, Van Houdenhove B, Bobbaers H. Does methylphenidate reduce the symptoms of chronic fatigue syndrome? *Am J Med*. 2006;119(2):167.e123-167.e130.

Bloomfield DM, ed. A common faint: tailoring treatment for targeted groups with vasovagal syncope. *Am J Cardiol*. 1999;84(8A):1Q-39Q.

Boehm KE, Kip KT, Grubb BP, Kosinski DJ. Neurocardiogenic syncope: response to hormonal therapy. *Pediatrics*. 1997;99(4):623-624.

Bonamichi-Santos R, Yoshimi-Kanamori K, Giavina-Bianchi P, Aun MV. Association of postural tachycardia syndrome and Ehlers–Danlos syndrome with mast cell activation disorders. *Immunol Allergy Clin North Am*. 2018;38(3):497-504.

Bou-Holaigah I, Calkins H, Flynn J, et al. Provocation of hypotension and pain during upright tilt table testing in adults with fibromyalgia. *Clin Exp Rheumatol*. 1997;15(3):239-246.

Bou-Holaigah I, Rowe PC, Kan J, Calkins H. The relationship between neurally mediated hypotension and the chronic fatigue syndrome. *JAMA*. 1995;274(12):961-967.

Brady PA, Low PA, Shen WK. Inappropriate sinus tachycardia, postural orthostatic tachycardia syndrome, and overlapping syndromes. *Pacing Clin Electrophysiol*. 2005;28(10):1112-1121.

Brignole M, Moya A, de Lange FJ, et al.; 2018 ESC Guidelines for the diagnosis and management of syncope. *Eur Heart J*. 2018;39(21):1883-1948.

Burklow TR, Moak JP, Bailey JJ, Makhlouf FT. Neurally mediated cardiac syncope: autonomic modulation after normal saline infusion. *J Am Coll Cardiol*. 1999;33(7):2059-2066.

Calkins H, Shyr Y, Frumin H, et al. The value of the clinical history in the differentiation of syncope due to ventricular tachycardia, atrioventricular block, and neurocardiogenic syncope. *Am J Med*. 1995;98:365-373.

Camfield PR, Camfield CS. Syncope in childhood: a case control clinical study of the familial tendency to faint. *Can J Neurol Sci*. 1990;17: 306-308.

Castori M, Morlino S, Ghibellini G, Celletti C, Camerota F, Grammatico P. Connective tissue, Ehlers–Danlos syndrome(s), and head and cervical pain. *Am J Med Genet C Semin Med Genet*. 2015;169(1):84-96.

Chan SM, Chodakiewitz YG, Maya MM, et al. Intracranial hypotension and cerebrospinal fluid leak. *Neuroimaging Clin N Am*. 2019;29(2): 213-226.

Chapman EM, Asmussen E. On the occurrence of dyspnea, dizziness and precordial distress occasioned by the pooling of blood in varicose veins. *J Clin Invest.* 1942;21(4):393–399.

Chobanian AV, Volicer L, Tifft CP, et al. Mineralocorticoid-induced hypertension in patients with orthostatic hypotension. *N Engl J Med.* 1979;301:68–73.

Coffin ST, Black BK, Biaggioni I, et al. Desmopressin acutely decreases tachycardia and improves symptoms in the postural tachycardia syndrome. *Heart Rhythm.* 2012;9(9):1484–1490.

Dani M, Dirksen A, Taraborrelli P, et al. Autonomic dysfunction in 'long COVID': rationale, physiology and management strategies. *Clin Med (Lond).* 2021;21(1):e63–e67.

de Cássia Collaço R, Lammens M, Blevins C, et al. Anxiety and dysautonomia symptoms in patients with a NaV1.7 mutation and the potential benefits of low-dose short-acting guanfacine. *Clin Auton Res.* 2023;34(1):191–201.

De Wandele I, Calders P, Peersman W, et al. Autonomic symptom burden in the hypermobility type of Ehlers–Danlos syndrome: a comparative study with two other EDS types, fibromyalgia, and healthy controls. *Semin Arthritis Rheum.* 2014;44(3):353–361.

De Wandele I, Rombaut L, De Backer T, et al. Orthostatic intolerance and fatigue in the hypermobility type of Ehlers–Danlos syndrome. *Rheumatology (Oxford).* 2016;55(8):1412–1420.

De Wandele I, Rombaut L, Leybaert L, et al. Dysautonomia and its underlying mechanisms in the hypermobility type of Ehlers–Danlos syndrome. *Semin Arthritis Rheum.* 2014;44(1):93–100.

Di Girolamo E, Di Iorio C, Sabatini P, et al. Effects of paroxetine hydrochloride, a selective serotonin reuptake inhibitor, on refractory vasovagal syncope: a randomized, double-blind, placebo-controlled study. *JACC.* 1999;33(5):1227–1230.

Edwards CC III, Edwards CC II, Heinlein S, et al. Case report: Recurrent cervical spinal stenosis masquerading as myalgic encephalomyelitis/chronic fatigue syndrome with orthostatic intolerance. *Front Neurol.* 2023;14:1284062.

Fanciulli A, Campese N, Wenning GK. The Schellong test: detecting orthostatic blood pressure and heart rate changes in German-speaking countries. *Clin Auton Res.* 2019;29(4):363–366.

Fedorowski A, Li H, Yu X, et al. Antiadrenergic autoimmunity in postural tachycardia syndrome. *Europace.* 2017;19(7):1211–1219.

Filler G, Gow RM, Nadarajah R, et al. Pharmacokinetics of pyridostigmine in a child with postural tachycardia syndrome. *Pediatrics.* 2006;118: e1563–e1568.

Fortunato JE, Shaltout HA, Larkin MM, et al. Fludrocortisone improves nausea in children with orthostatic intolerance (OI). *Clin Auton Res.* 2011;21:419-423.

Freeman R, Wieling W, Axelrod FB, et al. Consensus statement on the definition of orthostatic hypotension, neurally mediated syncope and the postural tachycardia syndrome. *Clin Auton Res.* 2011;21(2):69-72.

Goldstein DS. Post-COVID dysautonomias: what we know and (mainly) what we don't know. *Nature Reviews.* 2024;20(2):99-113.

Goldstein DS, Holmes C, Frank SM, et al. Cardiac sympathetic dysautonomia in chronic orthostatic intolerance syndromes. *Circulation.* 2002;106(18): 2358-2365.

Grubb BP. Neurocardiogenic syncope. *N Engl J Med.* 2005;352:1004-1010.

Grubb BP. Postural tachycardia syndrome. *Circulation.* 2008;117:2814-2817.

Grubb BP, Kosinski D, Mouhaffel A, Pothoulakis A. The use of methylphenidate in the treatment of refractory neurocardiogenic syncope. *PACE.* 1996; 19(5):836-840.

Grubb BP, Olshansky B, eds. *Syncope: Mechanisms and Management.* 2nd ed. Malden, MA: Blackwell Publishing; 2005.

Grubb BP, Wolfe DA, Samoil D, et al. Usefulness of fluoxetine hydrochloride for prevention of resistant upright tilt induced syncope. *PACE.* 1993;16:458-464.

Hall JE, Hall ME. *Guyton and Hall Textbook of Medical Physiology,* 14th ed. Philadelphia, PA: Elsevier; 2021.

Heffez DS, Ross RE, Shade-Zeldow Y, et al. Clinical evidence for cervical myelopathy due to Chiari malformation and spinal stenosis in a non-randomized group of patients with the diagnosis of fibromyalgia. *Eur Spine J.* 2004;13(6):516-523.

Heffez DS, Ross RE, Shade-Zeldow Y, et al. Treatment of cervical myelopathy in patients with the fibromyalgia syndrome: outcomes and implications. *Eur Spine J.* 2007;16(9):1423-1433.

Henderson FC, Sr., Rowe PC, Narayanan M, et al. Refractory syncope and presyncope associated with atlantoaxial instability: preliminary evidence of improvement following surgical stabilization. *World Neurosurg.* 2021;149:e854-e865.

Henderson FC, Sr., Schubart JR, Narayanan MV, et al. Craniocervical instability in patients with Ehlers-Danlos syndromes: outcomes analysis following occipito-cervical fusion. *Neurosurg Rev.* 2024;47(1):27.

Hyatt KH, Jacobson LB, Schneider VS. Comparison of 70 degrees tilt, LBNP, and passive standing as measures of orthostatic tolerance. *Aviat Space Environ Med.* 1975;46(6):801-808.

Institute of Medicine. *Beyond Myalgic Encephalomyelitis/Chronic Fatigue Syndrome: Redefining an Illness.* Washington, DC: National Academies Press; 2015.

Johnson JN, Mack KJ, Kuntz NL, Brands CK, Porter CJ, Fischer PR. Postural orthostatic tachycardia syndrome: a clinical review. *Pediatr Neurol.* 2010;42(2):77–85.

Jones MR, Prabhakar A, Viswanath O, et al. Thoracic outlet syndrome: a comprehensive review of pathophysiology, diagnosis, and treatment. *Pain Ther.* 2019;8(1):5–18.

Kanjwal K, Jamal S, Kichloo A, Grubb BP. New-onset postural orthostatic tachycardia syndrome following coronavirus disease 2019 infection. *J Innov Card Rhythm Manag.* 2020;11(11):4302–4304.

Kanjwal K, Karabin B, Kanjwal Y, Grubb BP. Outcomes of pregnancy in patients with preexisting postural tachycardia syndrome. *Pacing Clin Electrophysiol.* 2009;32(8):1000–1003.

Kanjwal K, Saeed B, Karabin B, Kanjwal Y, Grubb BP. Use of methylphenidate in the treatment of patients suffering from refractory postural tachycardia syndrome. *Am J Ther.* 2012;19(1):2–6.

Kaufmann H, Freeman R, Biaggioni I, et al. Droxidopa for neurogenic orthostatic hypotension: a randomized, placebo-controlled, phase 3 trial. *Neurology.* 2014;83(4):328–335.

Kelly KJ, Lazenby AJ, Rowe PC, Yardley JH, Perman JA, Sampson HA. Eosinophilic esophagitis attributed to gastroesophageal reflux: improvement with an amino acid-based formula. *Gastroenterology.* 1995;109: 1503–1512.

Kimpinski K, Iodice V, Sandroni P, Low PA. Effect of pregnancy on postural tachycardia syndrome. *Mayo Clin Proc.* 2010;85(7):639–644.

Knuttinen M-G, Zurcher KS, Khurana N, et al. Imaging findings of pelvic venous insufficiency in patients with postural orthostatic tachycardia syndrome. *Phlebology.* 2021;36(1):32–37.

Kokorelis C, Bodurtha J, Guthrie K, Rowe PC. Successful treatment of refractory orthostatic intolerance (OI) with droxidopa. *Clin Pediatr (Phila).* 2022;61(9):593–595.

Lewis T. A lecture on vasovagal syncope and the carotid sinus mechanism with comments on Gower's and Nothnagel's syndrome. *BMJ.* 1932; 873–876.

Li H, Yu X, Liles C, et al. Autoimmune basis for postural tachycardia syndrome. *J Am Heart Assoc.* 2014;3(1):e000755.

Low PA, Sandroni P, Joyner M, Shen WK. Postural tachycardia syndrome (POTS). *J Cardiovasc Electrophysiol.* 2009;20(3):352–358.

Mack KJ, Johnson JN, Rowe PC. Orthostatic intolerance and the headache patient. *Semin Pediatr Neurol.* 2010;17(2):109-116.

MacLean AR, Allen EV. Orthostatic hypotension and orthostatic tachycardia: treatment with the "head-up" bed. *JAMA.* 1940;115:2162-2167.

MacLean AR, Allen EV, Magath TB. Orthostatic tachycardia and orthostatic hypotension: defects in the return of venous blood to the heart. *Am Heart J.* 1944;27(2):145-163.

Mahanonda N, Bhuripanyo K, Kangkagate C, et al. Randomized double-blind, placebo-controlled trial of oral atenolol in patients with unexplained syncope and positive upright tilt table test results. *Am Heart J.* 1995; 130(6):1250-1253.

Malanga GA, Landes P, Nadler SF. Provocative tests in cervical spine examination: historical basis and scientific analyses. *Pain Physician.* 2003;6(2): 199-205.

Malek S, Reinhold EJ, Pearce GS. The Beighton Score as a measure of generalised joint hypermobility. *Rheumatol Int.* 2021;41:1707-1716.

Malfait F, Francomano C, Byers P, et al. The 2017 international classification of the Ehlers–Danlos syndromes. *Am J Med Genet Part C (Semin Med Genet).* 2017;175C:8-26.

Manyari DE, Rose S, Tyberg JV, et al. Abnormal reflex venous function in patients with neuromediated syncope. *J Am Coll Cardiol.* 1996;27: 1730-1735.

Masuki S, Eisenach JH, Johnson CP, et al. Excessive heart rate response to orthostatic stress in postural tachycardia syndrome is not caused by anxiety. *J Appl Physiol.* 2007;102(3):896-903.

McCance RA. Experimental sodium chloride deficiency in man. *Nutr Rev.* 1990;48(3):145-147.

McDonald C, Frith J, Newton JL. Single centre experience of ivabradine in postural orthostatic tachycardia syndrome. *Europace.* 2011;13:427-430.

Miglis MG, Prieto T, Shaik R, Muppidi S, Sinn D-I, Jaradeh S. A case report of postural tachycardia syndrome after COVID-19. *Clin Auton Res.* 2020;30(5):449-451.

Milhorat TH, Chou MW, Trinidad EM, et al. Chiari I malformation redefined: clinical and radiographic findings for 364 symptomatic patients. *Neurosurgery.* 1999;44(5):1005-1017.

Moak JP, Leong D, Fabian R, et al. Intravenous hydration for management of medication-resistant orthostatic intolerance in the adolescent and young adult. *Pediatr Cardiol.* 2016;37(2):278-282.

Moak JP, Ramwell C, Fabian R, Hanumanthaiah S, Darbari A, Kane TD. Median arcuate ligament syndrome with orthostatic intolerance:

intermediate-term outcomes following surgical intervention. *J Pediatr*. 2021;231:141–147.

Molderings GJ, Brettner S, Homann J, Afrin LB. Mast cell activation disease: a concise practical guide for diagnostic workup and therapeutic options. *J Hematol Oncol*. 2011;4:10.

National Academies of Sciences, Engineering, and Medicine. *Dietary Reference Intakes for Sodium and Potassium*. Washington, DC: National Academies Press; 2019.

Olson LG, Ambrogetti A, Sutherland DC. A pilot randomized controlled trial of dexamphetamine in patients with chronic fatigue syndrome. *Psychosomatics*. 2003;44(1):38–43.

Ozçakar L, Ertan H, Kaymak B. Two cases and two particular signs of thoracic outlet syndrome: tremor and tachycardia. *Rheumatol Int*. 2008;29(2): 227–228.

Park J, Didi M, Blair J. The diagnosis and treatment of adrenal insufficiency during childhood and adolescence. *Arch Dis Child*. 2016;101(9): 860–865.

Petracek LS, Broussard CA, Swope RL, Rowe PC. A case study of successful application of the principles of ME/CFS care to an individual with long COVID. *Healthcare*. 2023;11(6):865.

Petracek LS, Eastin EF, Rowe IR, Rowe PC. Orthostatic intolerance as a potential contributor to prolonged fatigue and inconsistent performance in elite swimmers. *BMC Sports Sci Med Rehabil*. 2022;14(1):139.

Petracek LS, Suskauer SJ, Vickers RF, et al. Adolescent and young adult ME/CFS after confirmed or probable COVID-19. *Front Med*. 2021;29(8):668944.

Plash WB, Diedrich A, Biaggioni I, et al. Diagnosing postural tachycardia syndrome: comparison of tilt testing compared with standing haemodynamics. *Clin Sci (Lond)*. 2012;124:109–114.

Platts SH, Tuxhorn JA, Ribeiro LC, Stenger MB, Lee SM, Meck JV. Compression garments as countermeasures to orthostatic intolerance. *Aviat Space Environ Med*. 2009;80(5):437–442.

Prilipko O, Dehdashti AR, Zaim S, Seeck M. Orthostatic intolerance and syncope associated with Chiari type I malformation. *J Neurol Neurosurg Psychiatry*. 2005;76(7):1034–1036.

Qingyou Z, Junbao D, Chaoshu T, et al. The efficacy of midodrine in the treatment of children with vasovagal syncope. *J Pediatr*. 2006;149(6): 777–780.

Raj SR, Black BK, Biaggioni I, Harris PA, Robertson D. Acetylcholinesterase inhibition improves tachycardia in postural tachycardia syndrome. *Circulation*. 2005;111:2734–2740.

Raj SR, Bourne KM, Stiles LE, et al. Postural orthostatic tachycardia syndrome (POTS): Priorities for POTS care and research from a 2019 National Institutes of Health Expert Consensus Meeting - Part 2. *Auton Neurosci.* 2021;235:102836.

Raj V, Haman KL, Raj SR, et al. Psychiatric profile and attention deficits in postural tachycardia syndrome. *J Neurol Neurosurg Psychiatry.* 2009;80(3):339-344.

Robertson D, Goldberg MR, Hollister AS, Wade D, Robertson RM, et al. Clonidine raises BP in severe idiopathic orthostatic hypotension. *Am J Med.* 1983;74(2):193-200.

Robinson SC. Hypotension: the ideal normal blood pressure. *N Engl J Med.* 1940;233:407-416.

Roma M, Marden CL, De Wandele I, Francomano CA, Rowe PC. Postural tachycardia syndrome and other forms of orthostatic intolerance in Ehlers-Danlos syndrome. *Auton Neurosci.* 2018;215:89-96.

Roma M, Marden CL, Flaherty MAK, Jasion SE, Cranston EM, Rowe PC. Impaired health-related quality of life in adolescent myalgic encephalomyelitis/chronic fatigue syndrome: the impact of core symptoms. *Front Pediatr.* 2019;7:26.

Roma M, Marden CL, Rowe PC. Passive standing tests for the office diagnosis of postural tachycardia syndrome: new methodological considerations. *Fatigue.* 2018;6(4):179-192.

Rosen SG, Cryer PE. Postural tachycardia syndrome: reversal of sympathetic hyperresponsiveness and clinical improvement during sodium loading. *Am J Med.* 1982;72:847-850.

Ross AJ, Medow MS, Rowe PC, et al. What is brain fog? An evaluation of the symptom in postural tachycardia syndrome. *Clin Auton Res.* 2013;23: 305-311.

Rowe KS. Long term follow up of young people with chronic fatigue syndrome attending a pediatric outpatient service. *Front Pediatr.* 2019;7:21.

Rowe PC, Barron DF, Calkins H, Maumenee IH, Tong PY, Geraghty MT. Orthostatic intolerance and chronic fatigue syndrome associated with Ehlers-Danlos syndrome. *J Pediatr.* 1999;135(4):494-499.

Rowe PC, Bou-Holaigah I, Kan JS, Calkins HG. Is neurally mediated hypotension an unrecognized cause of chronic fatigue? *Lancet.* 1995;345: 623-624.

Rowe PC, Calkins H, DeBusk K, et al. Fludrocortisone acetate to treat neurally mediated hypotension in chronic fatigue syndrome: a randomized controlled trial. *JAMA.* 2001;285(1):52-59.

Rowe PC, Fontaine KR, Lauver M, et al. Neuromuscular strain increases symptom intensity in chronic fatigue syndrome. *PLoS One*. 2016;11(7): e0159386.

Rowe PC, Fontaine KR, Violand RL. Neuromuscular strain as a contributor to cognitive and other symptoms in chronic fatigue syndrome. *Front Physiol*. 2013;4:115.

Rowe PC, Marden CL, Flaherty MAK, et al. Impaired range of motion of limbs and spine in chronic fatigue syndrome. *J Pediatr*. 2014;165(2):360–366.

Rowe PC, Marden CL, Heinlein S, Edwards CC. Improvement of severe myalgic encephalomyelitis/chronic fatigue syndrome symptoms following surgical treatment of cervical spinal stenosis. *J Transl Med*. 2018;16:21.

Rowe PC, Marden CL, Jasion SE, Cranston EM, Flaherty MAK, Kelly KJ. Cow's milk protein intolerance in adolescents and young adults with chronic fatigue syndrome. *Acta Paediatr*. 2016;105(9):e412–e418.

Rowell L. *Human Cardiovascular Control*. New York, NY: Oxford University Press; 1992.

Ruzieh M, Baugh A, Dasa O, et al. Effects of intermittent intravenous saline infusions in patients with medication-refractory postural tachycardia syndrome. *J Interv Card Electrophysiol*. 2017;48(3):255–260.

Salman IM. Major autonomic neuroregulatory pathways underlying short- and long-term control of cardiovascular function. *Curr Hypertens Rep*. 2016;18(3):18.

Samoil D, Grubb BP. Neurally mediated syncope and serotonin reuptake inhibitors. *Clin Auton Res*. 1999;5:251–255.

Sandmann W, Scholbach T, Verginis K. Surgical treatment of abdominal compression syndromes: the significance of hypermobility-related disorders. *Am J Med Genet C Semin Med Genet*. 2021;187(4):570–578.

Schondorf R, Low PA. Idiopathic postural orthostatic tachycardia syndrome: an attenuated form of acute pandysautonomia? *Neurology*. 1993;43: 132–137.

Sheldon RS, Faris P, Tang A, et al. Midodrine for the prevention of vasovagal syncope: a randomized clinical trial. *Ann Int Med*. 2021;174:1349–1356.

Sheldon RS, Grubb BP, Olshansky B, et al. 2015 Heart Rhythm Society expert consensus statement on the diagnosis and treatment of postural tachycardia syndrome, inappropriate sinus tachycardia, and vasovagal syncope. *Heart Rhythm*. 2015;12(6):e41–e63.

Sheldon RS, Raj SR, Rose MS, et al. Fludrocortisone for the prevention of vasovagal syncope: a randomized, placebo-controlled trial. *J Am Coll Cardiol*. 2016;68:1–9.

Shen WK, Sheldon RS, Benditt DG, et al. 2017 ACC/AHA/HRS guideline for the evaluation and management of patients with syncope: a report of the American College of Cardiology/American Heart Association Task Force on Clinical Practice Guidelines and the Heart Rhythm Society. *Heart Rhythm*. 2017;14:e155–e217.

Shibao C, Arzubiaga C, Roberts LJ, et al. Hyperadrenergic postural tachycardia syndrome in mast cell activation disorders. *Hypertension*. 2005;45(3): 385–390.

Shorter E. *From Paralysis to Fatigue: A History of Psychosomatic Illness in the Modern Era*. New York: Macmillan; 1992.

Singer W, Opfer-Gehrking TL, Nickander KK, Hines SM, Low PA. Acetylcholinesterase inhibition in patients with orthostatic intolerance. *J Clin Neurophysiol*. 2006;23(5):477–482.

Smit AA, Hardjowijono MA, Wieling W. Are portable folding chairs useful to combat orthostatic hypotension? *Ann Neurol*. 1997;42:975–978.

Smit AA, Wieling W, Fujimura J, et al. Use of lower abdominal compression to combat orthostatic hypotension in patients with autonomic dysfunction. *Clin Auton Res*. 2004;14:167–175.

Smith SJ, Sichlau MJ, Smith BH, Knight DRT, Chen B, Rowe PC. Improvement in chronic pelvic pain, orthostatic intolerance and interstitial cystitis symptoms after treatment of pelvic vein insufficiency. *Phlebology*. 2024;39(3):202–213

Stewart JM. Chronic orthostatic intolerance and the postural tachycardia syndrome (POTS). *J Pediatr*. 2004;145:725–730.

Stewart JM, Boris JR, Chelimsky G, et al. Pediatric disorders of orthostatic intolerance. *Pediatrics*. 2018;141(1):e20171673.

Stewart JM, Javaid S, Fialkoff T, et al. Initial orthostatic hypotension causes (transient) postural tachycardia. *J Am Coll Cardiol*. 2019;74(9):1271–1273.

Streeten DH, Thomas D, Bell DS. The roles of orthostatic hypotension, orthostatic tachycardia, and subnormal erythrocyte volume in the pathogenesis of the chronic fatigue syndrome. *Am J Med Sci*. 2000;320(1):1–8.

Sulheim D, Fagermoen E, Winger A, et al. Disease mechanisms and clonidine treatment in adolescent chronic fatigue syndrome: a combined cross-sectional and randomized controlled trial. *JAMA Pediatr*. 2014;168(4): 351–360.

Sullivan SD, Hanauer J, Rowe PC, Barron DF, Darbari A, Oliva-Hemker M. Gastrointestinal symptoms associated with orthostatic intolerance. *JPGN*. 2005;40(4):425–428.

Sutton R, Salukhe TV, Franzen-Mcmanus A-C, et al. Ivabradine in treatment of sinus tachycardia mediated vasovagal syncope. *Europace*. 2014;16:284–288.

Tandan T, Giuffre M, Sheldon RS. Exacerbations of neurally mediated syncope associated with sertraline. *Lancet*. 1997;349:1145-1146.

Taub PR, Zadourian A, Lo HC, Ormiston CK, Golshan S, Hsu JC. Randomized trial of ivabradine in patients with hyperadrenergic postural orthostatic tachycardia syndrome. *J Am Coll Cardiol*. 2021;77(7):861-871.

Ten Harkel ADJ, van Lieshout JJ, Wieling W. Treatment of orthostatic hypotension with sleeping in the head-up tilt position, alone and in combination with fludrocortisone. *J Intern Med*. 1992;232(2):139-145.

Towheed A, Nesheiwat Z, Mangi MA, Karabin B, Grubb BP. Ivabradine in children with postural orthostatic tachycardia syndrome: a retrospective study. *Cardiol Young*. 2020;30(7):975-979.

US Department of Agriculture. FoodData central. Agricultural Research Service. https://fdc.nal.usda.gov. Published 2019.

van Campen CMC, Rowe PC, Visser FC. Cerebral blood flow is reduced in severe ME/CFS patients during mild orthostatic stress testing: an exploratory study at 20 degrees of head-up tilt testing. *Healthcare*. 2020;8(2):169.

van Campen CMC, Rowe PC, Visser FC. Compression stockings improve cardiac output and cerebral blood flow during tilt testing in myalgic encephalomyelitis/chronic fatigue syndrome (ME/CFS) patients: a randomized crossover trial. *Medicina*. 2022;58(1):51.

van Campen CMC, Rowe PC, Visser FC. Orthostatic symptoms and reductions in cerebral blood flow in long-haul COVID-19 patients: similarities with myalgic encephalomyelitis/chronic fatigue syndrome. *Medicina*. 2022;58:28.

van Campen CMC, Rowe PC, Visser FC. Reductions in cerebral blood flow can be provoked by sitting in severe Myalgic encephalomyelitis/chronic fatigue syndrome patients. *Healthcare*. 2020;8:394.

van Campen CMC, Verheugt FWA, Rowe PC, et al. Cerebral blood flow is reduced in ME/CFS during head-up tilt testing even in the absence of hypotension or tachycardia: a quantitative, controlled study using Doppler echography. *Clin Neurophysiol Pract*. 2020;5:50-58.

van Campen CMC, Verheugt FWA, Visser FC. Cerebral blood flow changes during tilt table testing in healthy volunteers, as assessed by Doppler imaging of the carotid and vertebral arteries. *Clin Neurophysiol Pract*. 2018;3:91-95.

van Lieshout JJ, Ten Harkel ADJ, Wieling W. Physical manoeuvres for combating orthostatic dizziness in autonomic failure. *Lancet*. 1992;339(8798):897-898.

Venbrux AC, Chang AH, Kim HS, et al. Pelvic congestion syndrome (pelvic venous incompetence): impact of ovarian and internal iliac embolotherapy on menstrual cycle and chronic pelvic pain. *J Vasc Interv Radiol*. 2002;13:171-178.

Venbrux AC, Lambert DL. Embolization of the ovarian veins as a treatment for patients with chronic pelvic pain caused by pelvic vein incompetence (pelvic congestion syndrome). *Curr Opin Obstet Gynecol.* 1999;11(4): 395–399.

Vernino S, Bourne KM, Stiles LE, et al. Postural orthostatic tachycardia syndrome (POTS): state of the science and clinical care from a 2019 National Institutes of Health Expert Consensus Meeting - part 1. *Auton Neurosci.* 2021;235:102828.

Warad DM, Rao AN, Bjarnason H, Rodriguez V. Clinical outcomes of May-Thurner syndrome in pediatric patients: a single institutional experience. *TH Open.* 2020;4(3):e189–e196.

Ward CR, Gray J, Gilroy J, Kenny R. Midodrine: a role in the management of neurocardiogenic syncope. *Heart.* 1998;79(1):45–49.

White KP, Speechley M, Harth M, et al. Co-existence of chronic fatigue syndrome with fibromyalgia syndrome in the general population: a controlled study. *Scand J Rheumatol.* 2000;29:44–51.

Wieling W, Krediet CTP, van Dijk N, et al. Initial orthostatic hypotension: review of a forgotten condition. *Clin Sci.* 2007;112:157–165.

Wieling W, Shepherd JT. Initial and delayed circulatory responses to orthostatic stress in normal humans and in subjects with orthostatic intolerance. *Int Angiol.* 1992;11(1):69–82.

Wieling W, van Lieshout JJ, van Leeuwen AM. Physical manoeuvres that reduce postural hypotension in autonomic failure. *Clin Auton Res.* 1993;3(1):57–65.

Wyller VB, Saul JP, Amlie JP, Thaulow E. Sympathetic predominance of cardiovascular regulation during mild orthostatic stress in adolescents with chronic fatigue. *Clin Physiol Funct Imaging.* 2007;27(4):231–238.

Young JL. Use of lisdexamfetamine dimesylate in treatment of executive functioning deficits and chronic fatigue syndrome: a double blind, placebo-controlled study. *Psychiatry Res.* 2013;207(1–2):127–133.

Zeng C, Zhu Z, Liu G, et al. Randomized, double-blind, placebo-controlled trial of oral enalapril in patients with neurally mediated syncope. *Am Heart J.* 1998;136(5):852–858.

INDEX